HEINEMANN CHILDREN'S REFERENCE
a division of Heinemann Educational Books Ltd
Halley Court, Jordan Hill, Oxford OX2 8EJ

OXFORD LONDON EDINBURGH
MELBOURNE SYDNEY AUCKLAND
MADRID ATHENS BOLOGNA
SINGAPORE IBADAN NAIROBI HARARE
GABORONE KINGSTON PORTSMOUTH NH(USA)

ISBN 0 431 00736 5

British Library Cataloguing in Publication Data
Steele, Philip
  Food and diet
  1. Food
  I. Title II. Series
  641.3

Designed by Julian Holland Publishing Ltd
Colour artwork by George Fryer
Picture research by Karen Gunnell

Printed in Hong Kong

91 92 93 94 95 96 10 9 8 7 6 5 4 3 2 1

Photographic credits
t = top *b* = bottom *l* = left *r* = right

Cover: Science Photo Library
2 Camerapix; 4*b* The Hutchison Library, 8*b* ALLSPORT Bob Martin;
9*b* Barnaby's Picture Library; 10*t* Weightwatchers; 10*b* The Hutchison
Library; 11*t* Mehta/Colourific!; 12*b* Tourism Division, TX Dept of
Commerce; 13*t*, 13*b* The Hutchison Library; 14*b* ZEFA; 15*t* Science
Photo Library/Phillipe Plailly; 15*b* ZEFA; 16*b* National Dairy Council;
17*t* Sally and Richard Greenhill; 17*b* Bowyers; 18*t* Bryan and Cherry
Alexander; 19*t* Birds Eye Wall's Ltd; 19*b*, 20*b* ZEFA; 21*t* Sally and
Richard Greenhill; 21*b* The Anthony Blake Photo Library; 22*b*, 23*t* Sally
and Richard Greenhill; 23*b* Braun; 24*t* The Hutchison Library; 25*t*
ICCE Mark Boulton; 25*b* Frank Spooner; 27*t* Ace Photo Library/Ronald
Toms; 27*b* Holt Studios Ltd; 28*b* Science Photo Library/Phillipe Plailly;
29*t* NASA/Science Photo Library; 30*b* The Hutchison Library

Note to the reader
In this book there are some words in the text which are printed in **bold** type. This shows that the word is listed in the glossary on page 31. The glossary gives a brief explanation of words which may be new to you.

FOOD and DIET

Philip Steele

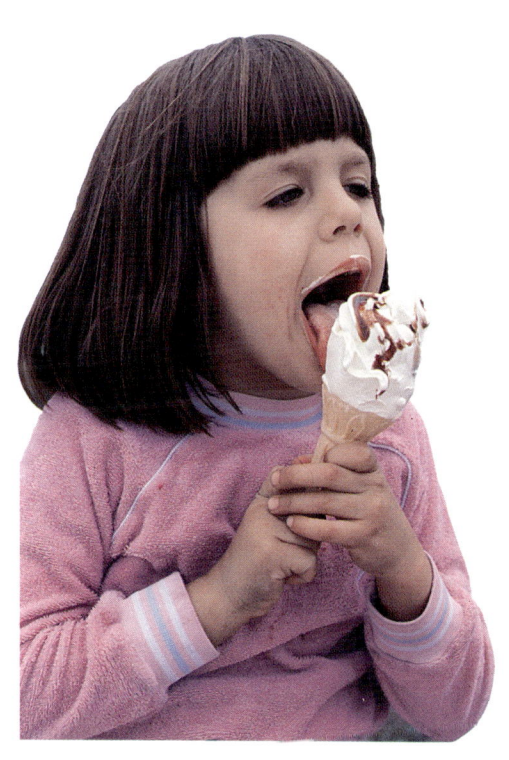

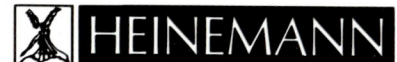

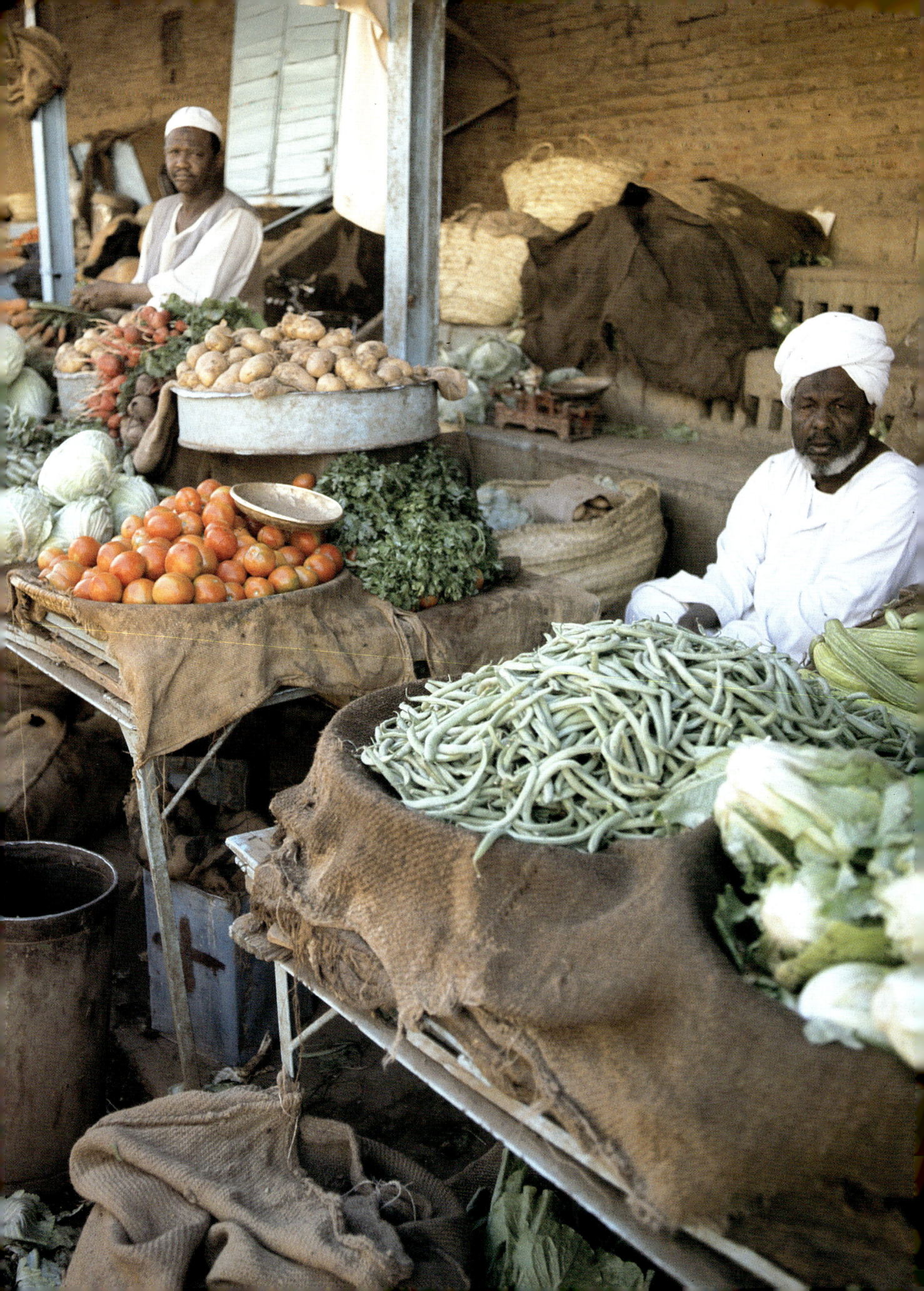

Contents

Food and the body

The human body turns the food we eat into the chemicals which fuel our bodies and keep us alive. They give us the energy to exercise, grow and stay healthy. This process is called **digestion**.

The body at work

As soon as someone sees a tasty meal, the production line inside their body gets ready. Chemicals are squirted into the mouth and stomach. They make the mouth water and the stomach rumble.

The food is put in the mouth, where the teeth chew it into small pieces. Saliva or spit is released into the mouth, and this makes the food easy to swallow. The food then passes into a tube called the oesophagus and is squeezed down into the stomach.

The stomach is a sort of bag designed to churn the food into a pulp. In the stomach the food is treated with acid. Chemicals called **enzymes** help to start the breakdown of the food into the various fuels used by the body. After at least a couple of hours in the stomach, the food is ready to move on.

It passes into a long, narrow tube called the small

▽ **A Chinese family in Beijing enjoy a meal together. We need food and water every day in order to live and to stay healthy.**

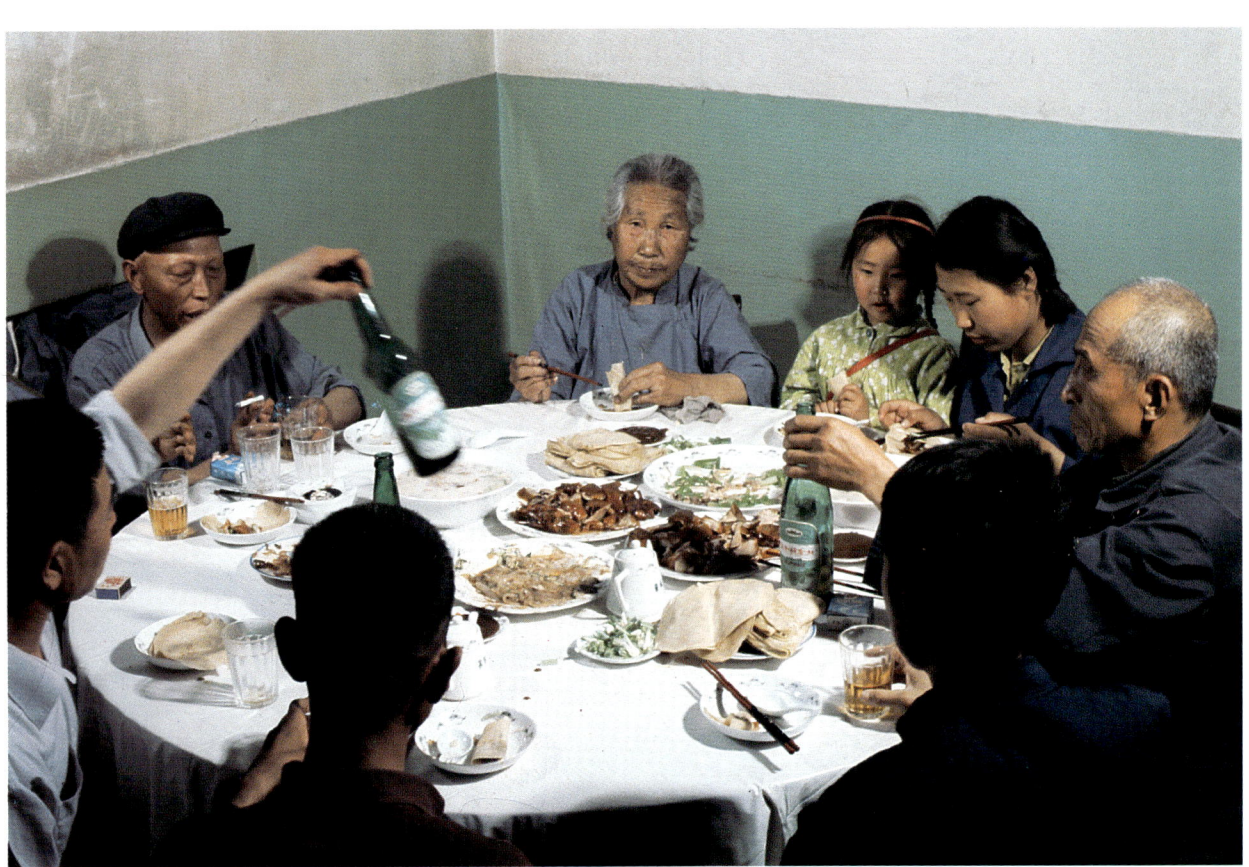

How we digest our food

Fuel intake Food is prepared for digestion in the mouth. It is chewed by teeth and saliva is added.

The tube Food is swallowed and passed down the oesophagus.

The acid bath The stomach breaks down the food with acids and other chemicals.

The digester The small intestine processes the food and passes it into the bloodstream.

The press The large intestine squeezes the food remains dry and passes any remaining goodness into the bloodstream.

The refinery The liver processes the body fuels once they have been passed into the bloodstream.

The exhaust Solid waste is stored in the rectum and then passed from the body.

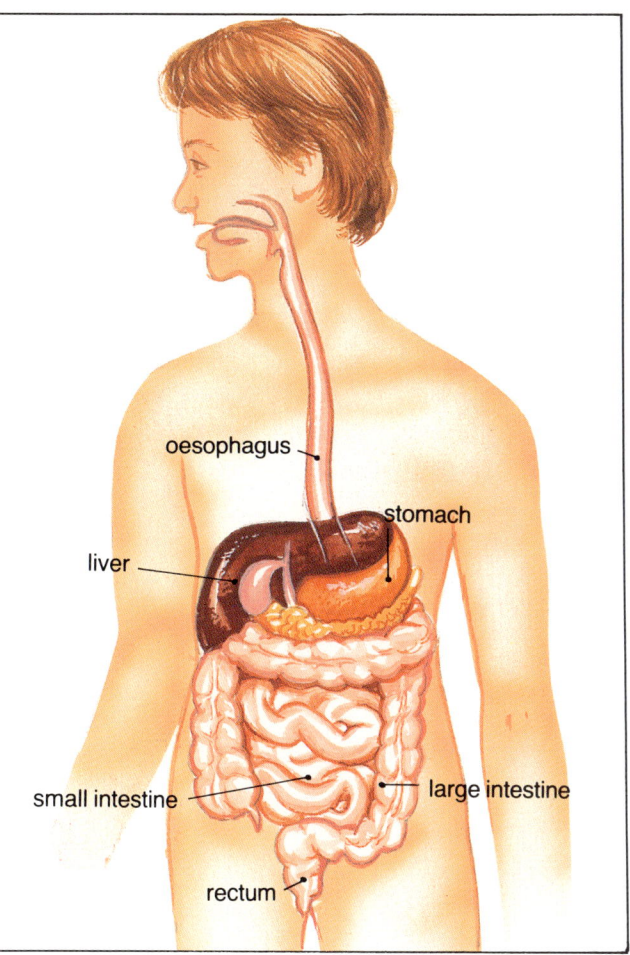

oesophagus

stomach

liver

small intestine

large intestine

rectum

intestine. There the food is squeezed and further chemicals are added. It turns from pulp into liquid. The inside of the small intestine is covered in bumps called villi. The surface area inside the intestine is about 20 square metres. Over the whole of this area, chemicals are passed from the food into the bloodstream, through the intestine wall. The enriched blood passes through the liver, where further processing takes place. Every part of the body can now receive life-giving fuels. Waste chemicals from the blood are filtered by the kidneys and passed from the body as a waste liquid called urine.

The remains of food which cannot be digested are now squeezed dry in the short, wide tube called the large intestine. The solid waste is passed from the body through the rectum.

Food and science
A car cannot run without fuel, and our bodies cannot work without food and water. This book examines the way in which food affects our health, and the way in which it is produced and processed. In a world in which many people are starving, the science of food is the science of survival.

What is food?

Human beings are able to eat both plants and animals as food. The first people spent every day searching for food and water. They picked wild berries and dug up roots. They ate insects and grubs, shellfish, and the raw flesh of the animals that they trapped and hunted.

Today, food is mostly produced by farmers, who grow crops and breed animals for food. Water is piped into our homes. Much of the food eaten has already been chopped and cooked and mixed in factories. We buy our food in tins and packets at the supermarket. Very few of us eat food that we have hunted or grown for ourselves.

Body fuels

In the last 200 years, the knowledge of food has become based on science. We now know which foods are good for us and which are bad. Food chemicals which can be turned into body fuel are called **nutrients.** Some of the most important nutrients are called **fats.** They are our main source of energy, and are found in meat, dairy products and plant oils. Too much animal fat can make us ill. Energy is also supplied by nutrients called **carbohydrates**. These are found in sugar, and also in bread, potatoes and **cereals**. **Proteins** too can supply us with energy. These nutrients are found in meat, fish, cheese and beans. Proteins help us grow, building up the tiny **cells** from which our bodies are made.

Our food contains other natural chemicals. Scientists have given names or letters to these **vitamins**, and found out which parts of the body they affect.

Other important nutrients are called **minerals**. Salt, iron, calcium and phosphorus are all minerals that keep us healthy. Iron, found in green vegetables, helps the blood carry life-giving oxygen around the body. Calcium from milk is good for our bones and teeth.

Water carries the nutrients from digested food into the bloodstream, which takes them to the cells where they are used for energy and growth. The water then carries the waste out of the body in the form of urine.

Non-fuels

Some parts of food are not used as body fuels, but carry out other useful functions. Fibre makes up the raw bulk of vegetables, fruit and cereals. It helps to exercise the muscles in the intestines.

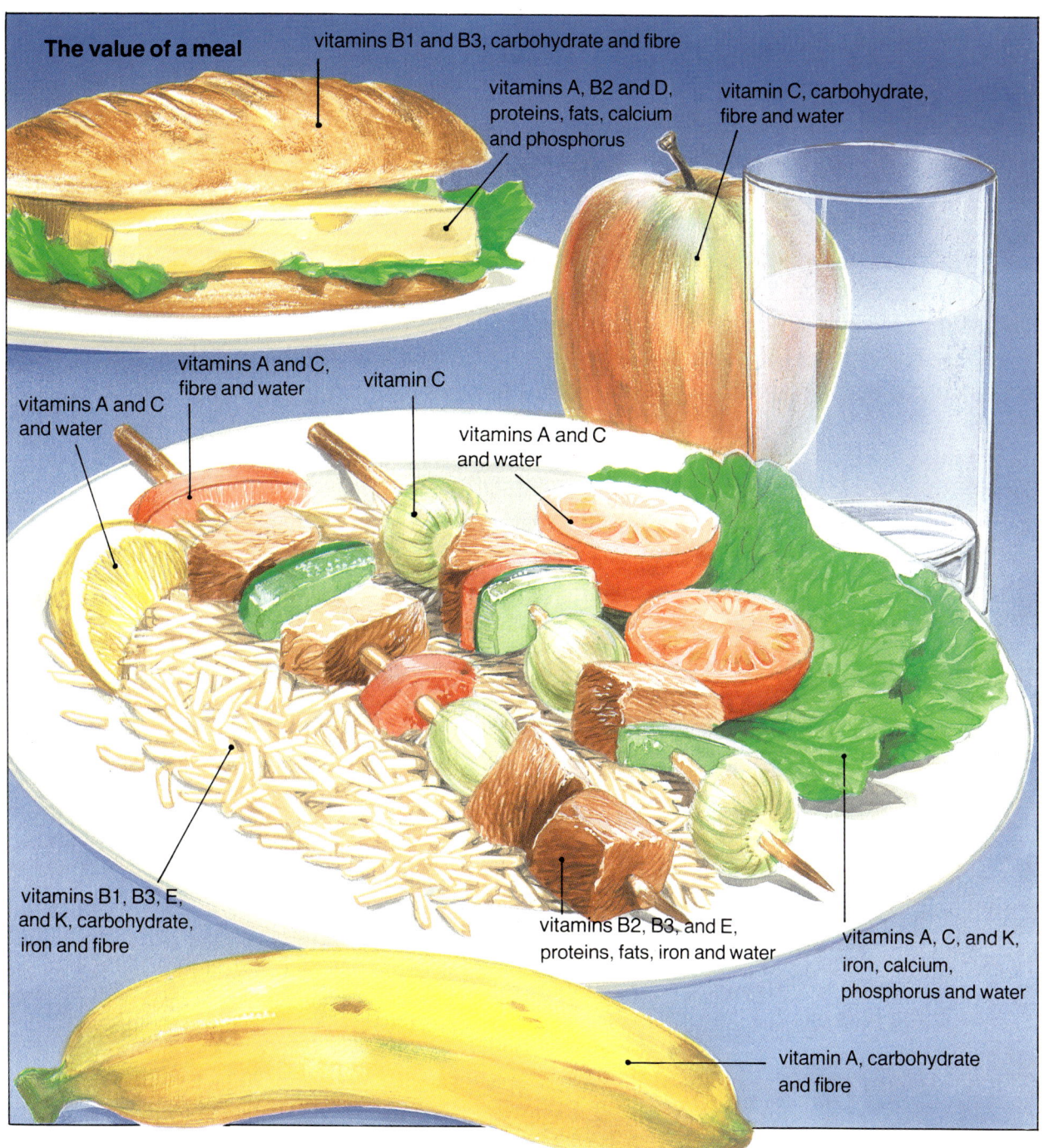

The value of a meal

vitamins B1 and B3, carbohydrate and fibre

vitamins A, B2 and D, proteins, fats, calcium and phosphorus

vitamin C, carbohydrate, fibre and water

vitamins A and C, fibre and water

vitamin C

vitamins A and C and water

vitamins A and C and water

vitamins B1, B3, E, and K, carbohydrate, iron and fibre

vitamins B2, B3, and E, proteins, fats, iron and water

vitamins A, C, and K, iron, calcium, phosphorus and water

vitamin A, carbohydrate and fibre

Vitamin A for skin, eyes, nose and throat	**Vitamin B1** for digestion	**Vitamin B2** for healthy skin	**Vitamin B3** for digestion and nerves
Vitamin C for gums, teeth and bones	**Vitamin D** for teeth and bones	**Vitamin E** for cell tissues	**Vitamin K** for clotting of blood
Proteins for growth	**Carbohydrates** for energy	**Fats** for growth and energy	**Fibre** to help the digestion
Water for cells and digestion	**Iron** for carrying oxygen in the blood	**Calcium and phosphorus** for bones and teeth	

Why we need to eat

The chemical factory inside our bodies turns nutrients into fuels. The fats are broken down to form **fatty acids.** These are stored in the body, and supply us with warmth and strength. Broken down fats also produce a chemical called **glycerol**, which stocks up our reserves of energy. Carbohydrates are broken down and turned into a sugary chemical called **glucose**. This too supplies us with energy. Enzymes break down proteins into chemicals called **amino acids**, which build up the body and keep it in good repair.

We need to eat for body growth, repair and energy. The kind of food we eat, or our diet, must be balanced. It must contain all the nutrients we need in the right amounts.

Shortage of food

If people take no water or food, they die. After only a couple of days without food, they begin to feel ill.

Many people in the world cannot get enough food to eat. They may be poor, or their crops may fail. The few scraps of food they do find cannot supply enough nutrients to keep the body healthy. Soon they begin to starve. Their bodies become weak and unable to resist disease.

▽ **Energy is created when glucose and amino acids react with oxygen in the body's cells. Exercise, such as a fast sprint, burns up the energy we get from food. It keeps us fit.**

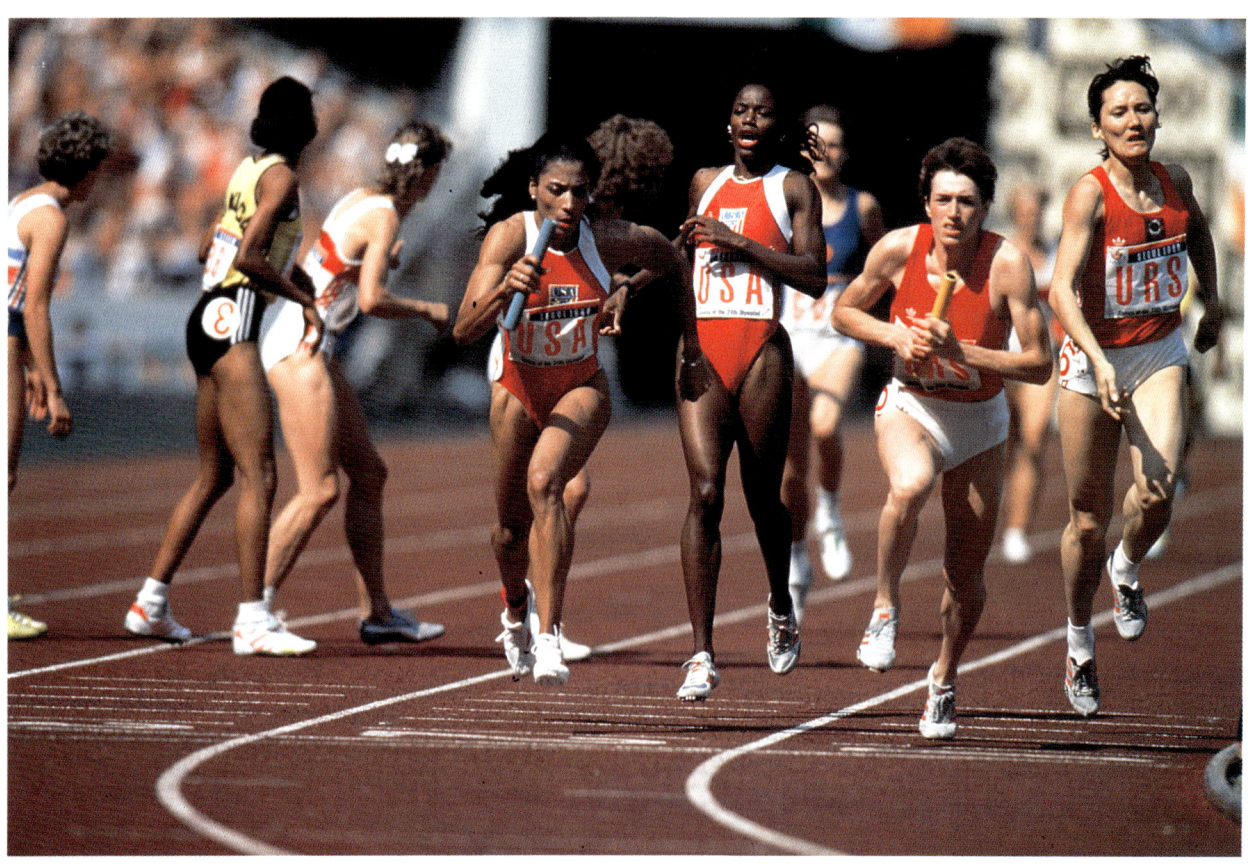

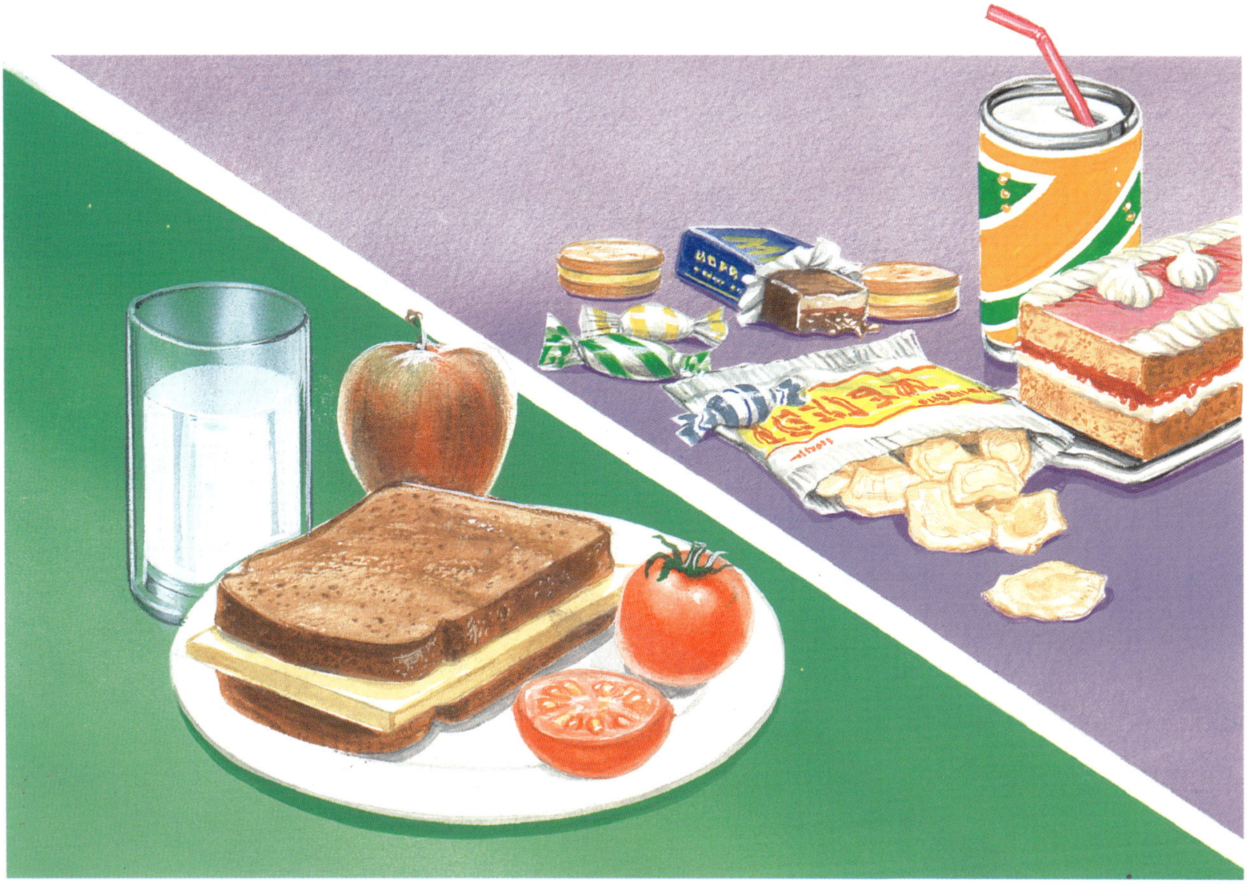

A lack of the right nutrients leads to **malnutrition**. With the wrong fuel mixture, the body begins to go wrong. A shortage of vitamin B1 can lead to the disease beri-beri. The arms and legs become very thin and the nerves in them no longer work properly. The stomach swells up and the victim feels very weak.

If children do not have enough vitamin D or calcium, their bones may soften and become deformed. This disease is called rickets. People who lack vitamin C in their diet may suffer from scurvy. Their skin becomes spotty and their gums bleed.

Too much food

Malnutrition is not only common in places where there are food shortages and poor people. Many people eat the wrong kinds of food, and make themselves ill. They may eat too much fatty food. This can give them heart disease. They may eat only soft, processed food. Without rough fibre to keep the intestine active, it can become distressed and stop working properly.

If people take little or no exercise, they do not use up enough energy. Their bodies store up too much unused fuel and they become fat. Having to carry around extra weight can strain the body and can also cause heart disease and other problems.

△ **A balanced diet** (left) includes a variety of fresh foods. Sweets and crisps alone (right) cannot supply the body with all the nutrients it needs.

▽ **Poor families** may not be able to buy enough food for their children. Constant hunger can lead to ill health, as well as problems with learning and patterns of behaviour.

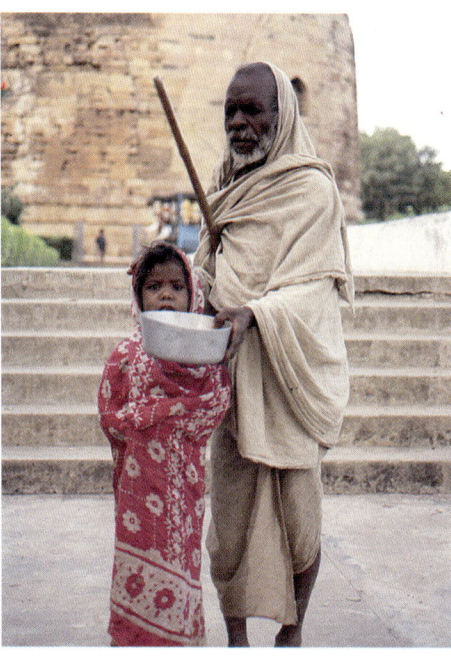

Diet control

The food we eat affects the way in which our bodies work. By controlling our diet, we can make ourselves healthier and stronger, or change the way we look.

Doctor's orders

Many people have to eat special food when they are ill. Some of them suffer from a disease called diabetes. Their bodies cannot make use of the sugar that they eat. They have to eat food which contains little or no sugar. Other people must avoid eating salt, and some people become ill if they eat eggs, flour or other items of food.

People who are weakened by illness or old age may need to be given pills containing vitamins, minerals or other nutrients. If people are already eating a balanced diet, such pills are not necessary.

Weight problems

The reason most people try a special diet is to lose weight. People who become fat through eating too much need to eat less food and healthier food. They must take more exercise to use up the energy provided by the food.

Like other kinds of energy, such as heat, food energy can be measured. Units of measurement used include kilogram calories (kcal) and kilojoules (kJ). A dieting chart might show that a boiled egg has 45 kcal (191kJ) while a fried egg has 70 kcal (298kJ). We can also check on how much energy we are using up in exercise. Charts show that playing football or hard cycling uses up 600 kcal (2550kJ) an hour.

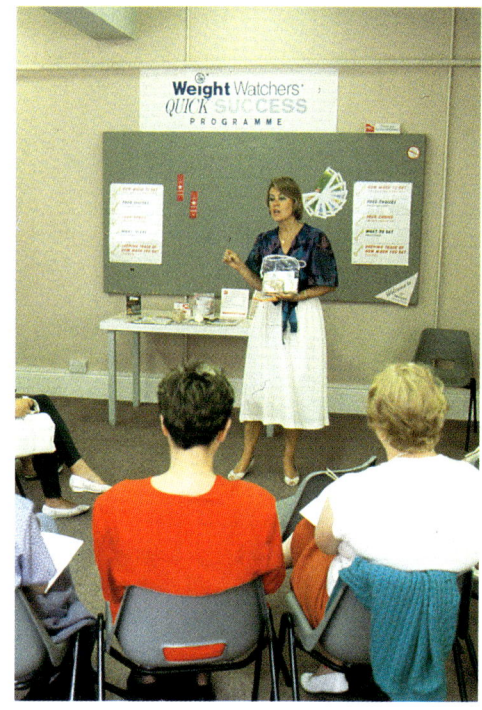

△ **Many special diets have been worked out to help people lose weight. Some overweight people meet regularly to discuss their problems. They encourage each other to eat less and take more exercise.**

▽ **Sports make special demands on the body. Athletes may choose a diet to lose weight or to gain weight, or to build up the muscles. Japanese Sumo wrestlers need to weigh about 135 kilograms to be successful.**

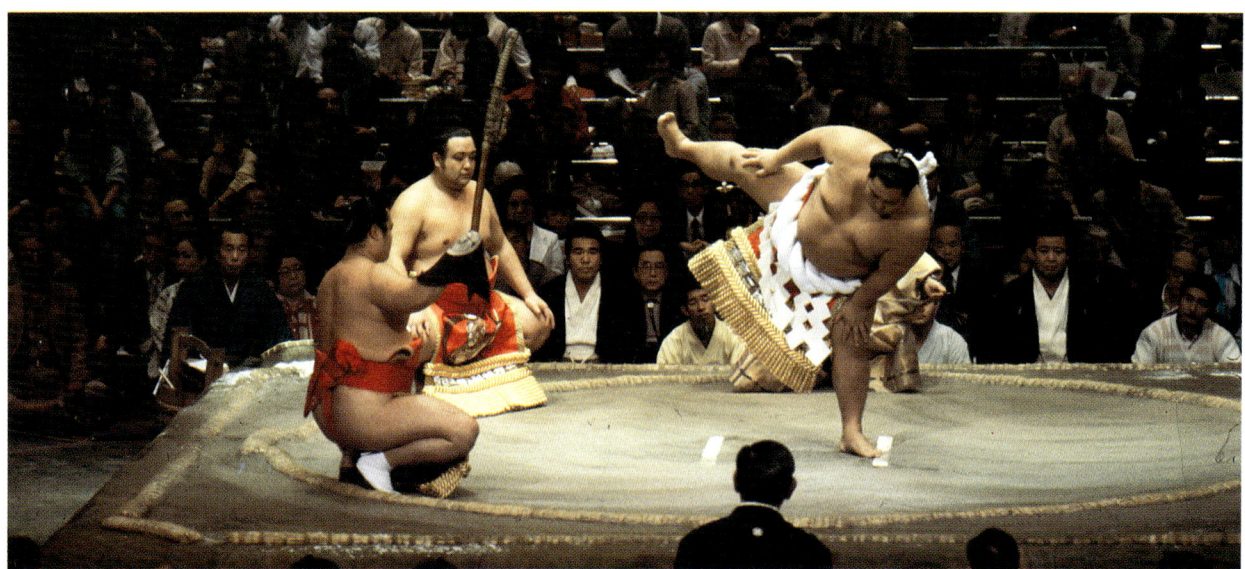

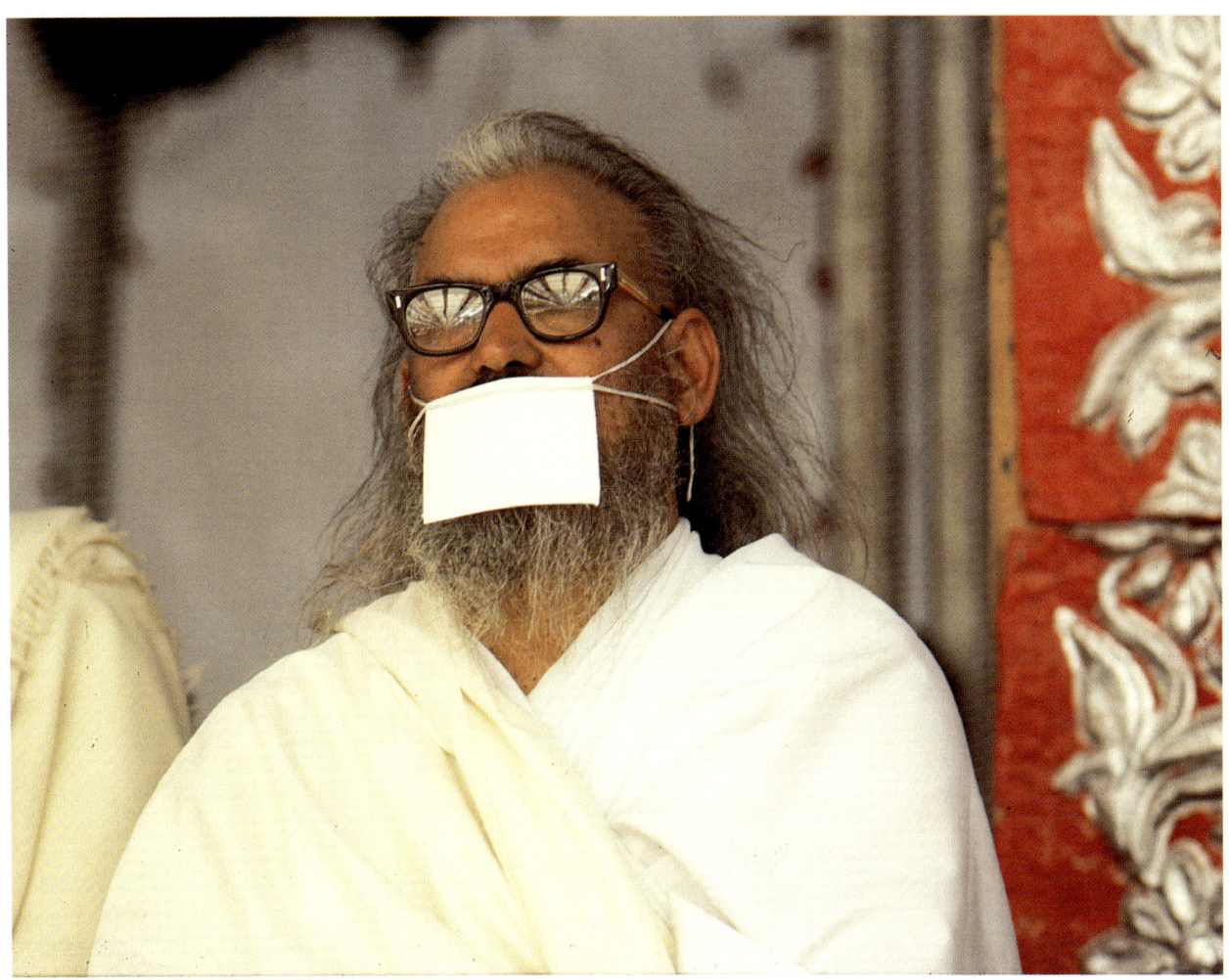

△ **Many religions have rules about diet. Jewish people may not eat pork. Hindus may not eat beef. This Jain priest is a strict vegetarian. He even wears a mask to prevent him swallowing a fly by mistake.**

People sometimes worry too much about their weight. They go on a special diet when they do not really need to. Some manufacturers play on these fears and advertise diets which are not suitable. Some young people become obsessed with dieting. They may suffer from an illness called anorexia nervosa, in which they lose all appetite for food. If you are going to diet, it is best to get medical advice. For most people, healthy food and plenty of exercise is quite enough to get into shape.

Eating no meat

Many people choose to eat only certain kinds of foods. Vegetarians will not eat meat. Vegans will not eat any kind of animal products, including eggs, cheese and milk. Some of them believe that we have no right to take the life of a fellow creature. Some think that modern farming methods are cruel to animals. Others believe that the raising of cattle and sheep is a wasteful way of using the world's resources. Meat-free diets are perfectly healthy provided that the body receives the right balance of nutrients from other sources.

Food from plants and animals

About 5000 million people live in the world today. Each of those people needs to eat about 50 tonnes of food during their lifetime. Most of that food will come from plants grown by farmers. In every part of the world there is one particular food, such as bread or rice, which is the basis of most people's diets. The plants providing such basic foods are called staple crops.

Crops for food

We eat all kinds of plants, and many different parts of those plants. We eat leaves, such as cabbage and lettuce. We eat flowers such as cauliflowers, and roots such as carrots. We eat the stems of celery and the swollen underground stems, or tubers, of the potato plant. We eat fruits such as apples, oranges and mangoes. Tomatoes and cucumbers are often called vegetables, but they are really fruits as well.

Seeds are one of the major food sources, providing carbohydrates for energy. The seeds of rice, wheat and maize are the most important cereals. Rice grows in hot countries such as India and China. Rice seedlings are planted in flooded fields and grown to a height of one metre or more. The fields are then drained and the grain is left to ripen. The crop is harvested and threshed.

▽ **Beef cattle provide us with a high-energy food source. A 200 gram steak contains 390 kcal (1638kJ). However, rearing cattle is expensive and takes up a lot of land that could be used for growing crops.**

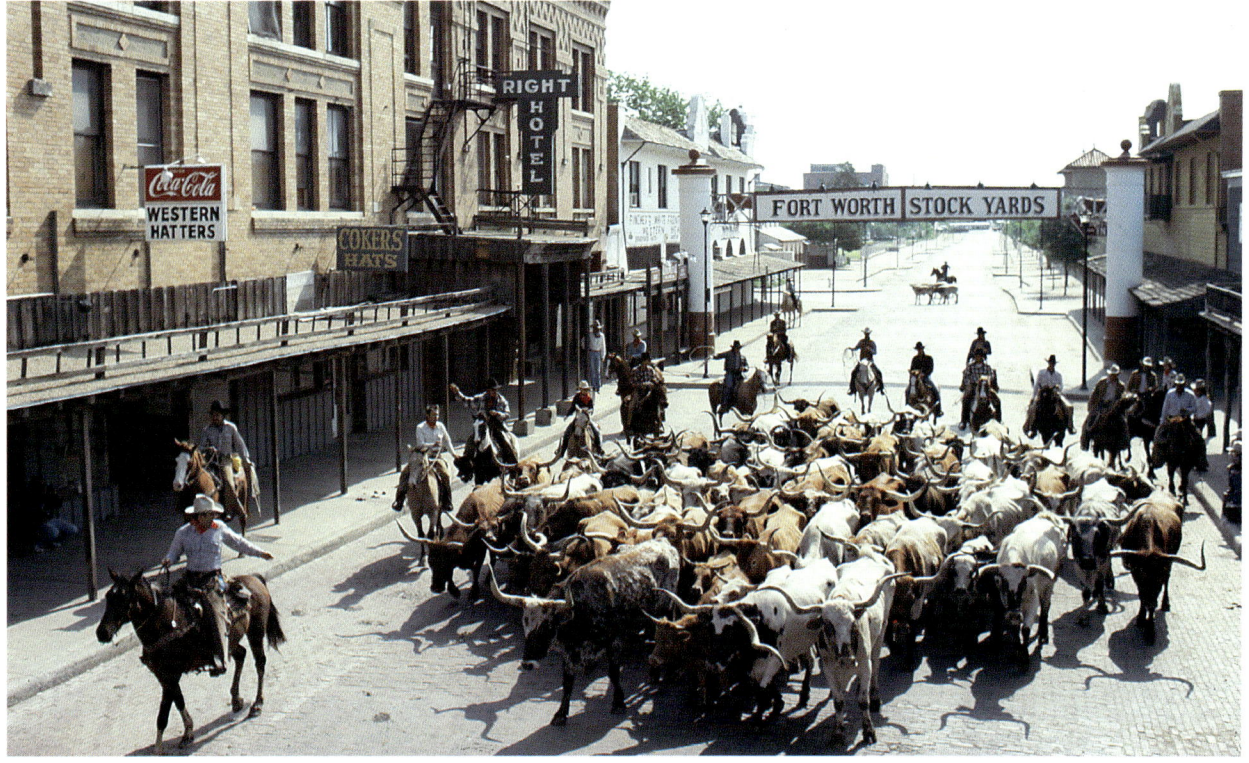

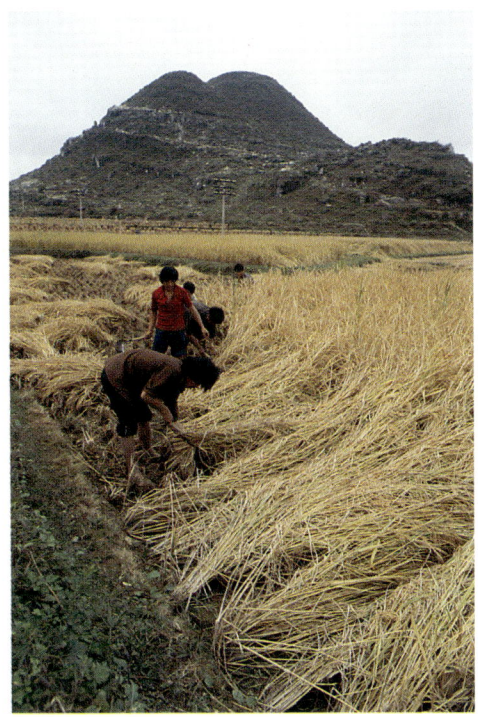

△ In Asia rice is normally harvested by hand. The rough grain is called paddy. It must be threshed and cleaned before it is ready to be cooked. Rice is a staple food for half the world's population.

The main wheat producers are the USSR, China and the United States. Wheat grows in dry soil, in regions with a colder climate. It is harvested and threshed, and ground into flour. The flour may be used to make bread or pasta. The female maize plant produces a large seed-head, or cob. This may be cooked, ground into cornflour, or used for making cornflakes and cooking oil.

Seeds such as peas, beans and lentils are known as **pulses**. They are a rich source of protein. Beans from the soya plant can be processed to make a food which looks like meat.

Oils for cooking and preparing foods can be obtained from seeds such as sunflower, from beans such as soya, and from fruits such as the olive.

Animals for food

Many different animals supply us with meat. Meat is the main source of protein in food. The most common meats are pork, lamb and beef. Milk is taken from cows, and also from goats and sheep. It can be turned into butter and cheese. Turkeys, ducks and chickens also provide us with meat, and their eggs are another protein source. Fish are rich in protein and vitamin D. They are taken from all the world's oceans and many of its lakes and rivers. Fish are also raised on fish farms.

▷ Thousands of Nigerians compete to catch Nile perch in this traditional fishing festival. In most African countries the diet is based on carbohydrates from cereals such as maize, or from tubers such as cassava. Fish add vital protein and vitamins to the diet.

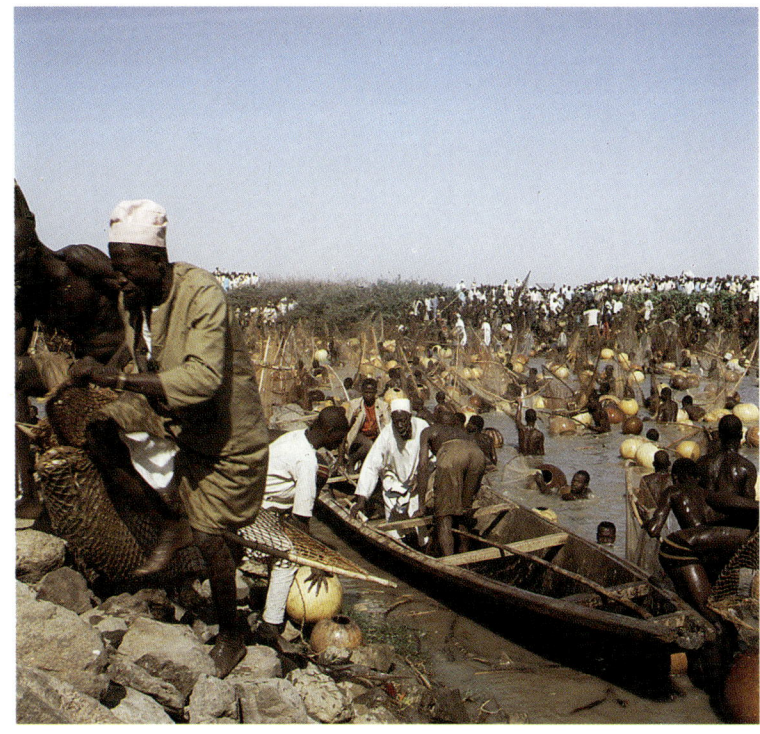

Science and the harvest

The first people to practise agriculture, or the growing of crops for food, lived about 11 000 years ago in the area known today as the Middle East. Later, farmers learned to tame wild animals and to breed them for food. From the very start, farming was at the forefront of developments in new science and technology.

People learned how to plough and sow. They learned how to dig channels through the desert, carrying precious water for the **irrigation** of crops. They learned how to **fertilize** the land, making it rich by spreading it with animal dung. They learned how to improve strains of crops. The best quality grain was not eaten but saved for sowing the following spring.

A new age

From the beginning of the 17th century, farming became more and more technological. Scientists learned how the characteristics of plants and animals are passed on from one generation to the next. They learned how to cross two different kinds of plant to produce a **hybrid**. Factories produced new chemicals to enrich the soil. Engineers designed new machines to harvest and thresh cereal crops.

In more recent times, many farms have been organized

▽ **Harvesting used to be back-breaking work. Today, combine harvesters cut and thresh wheat in one operation.**

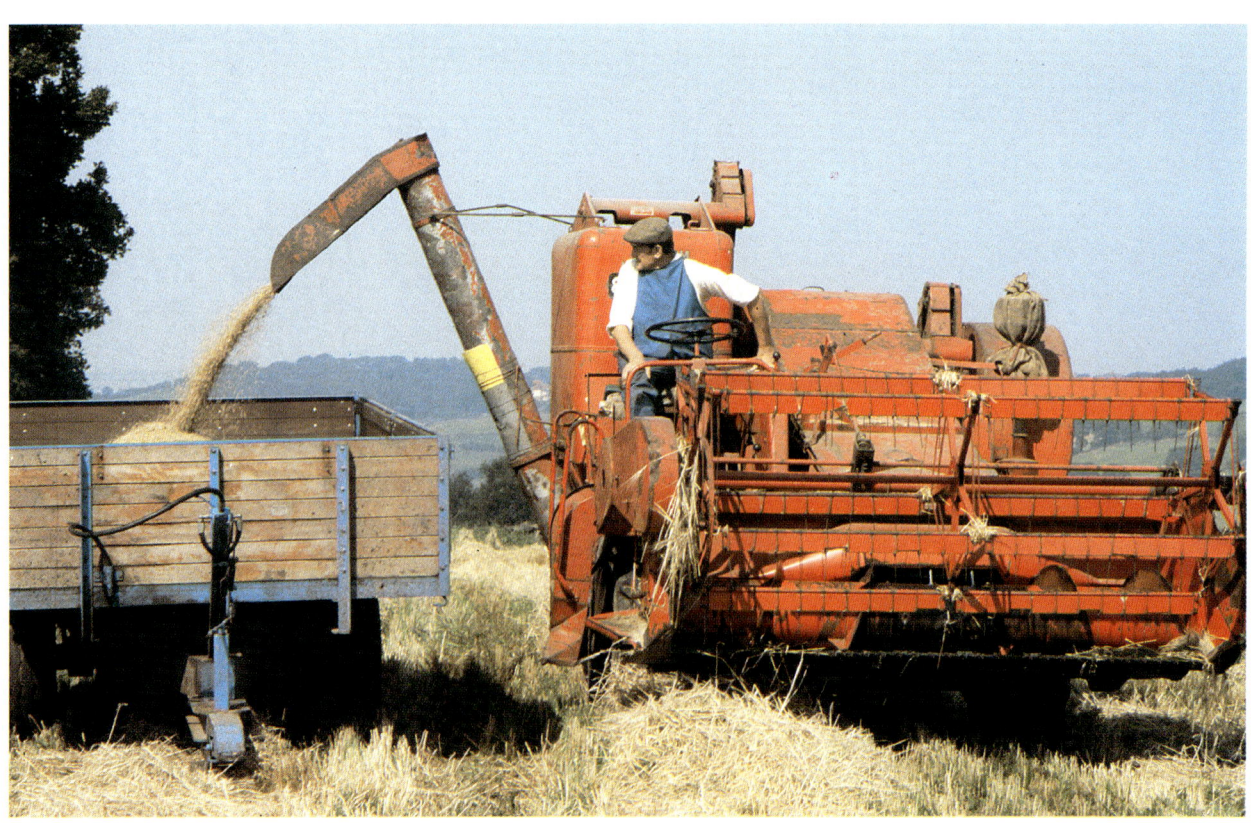

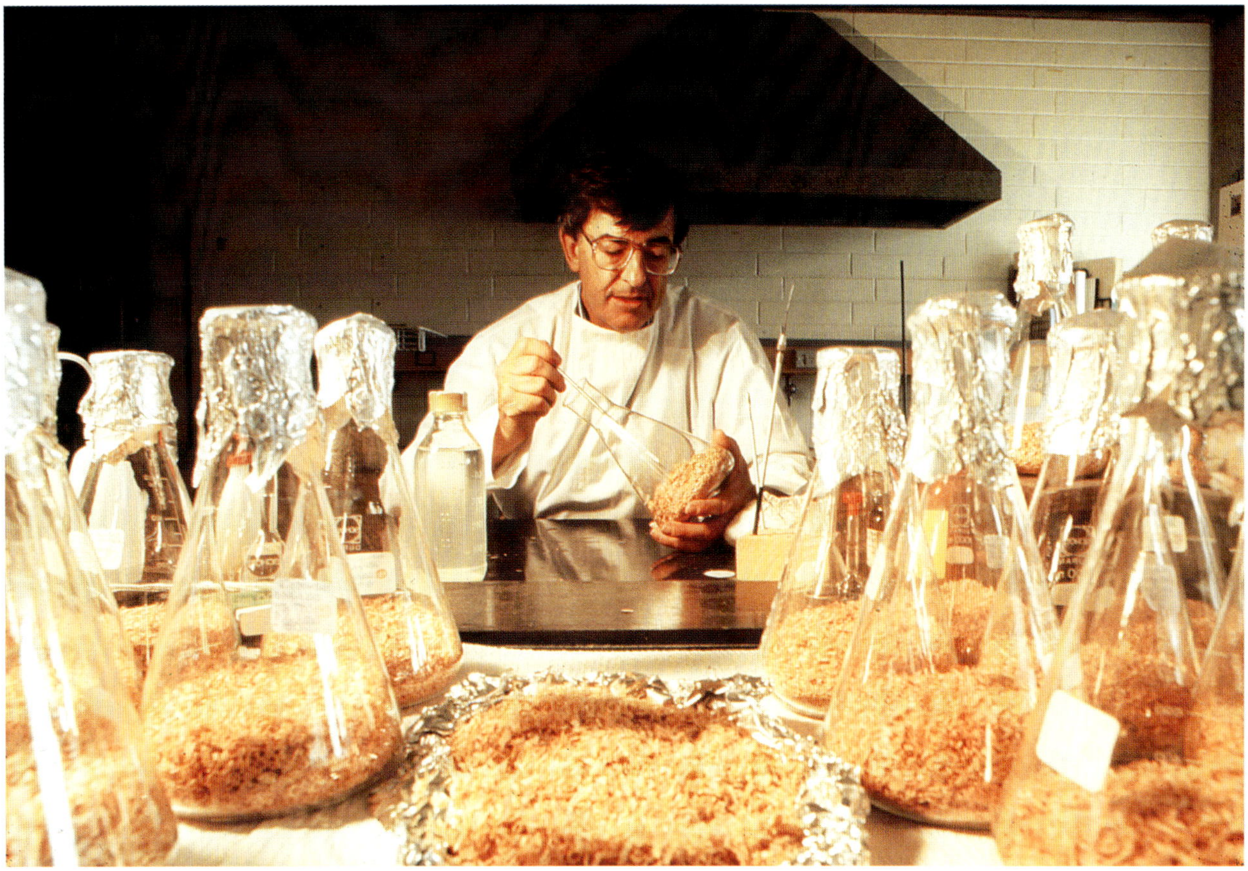

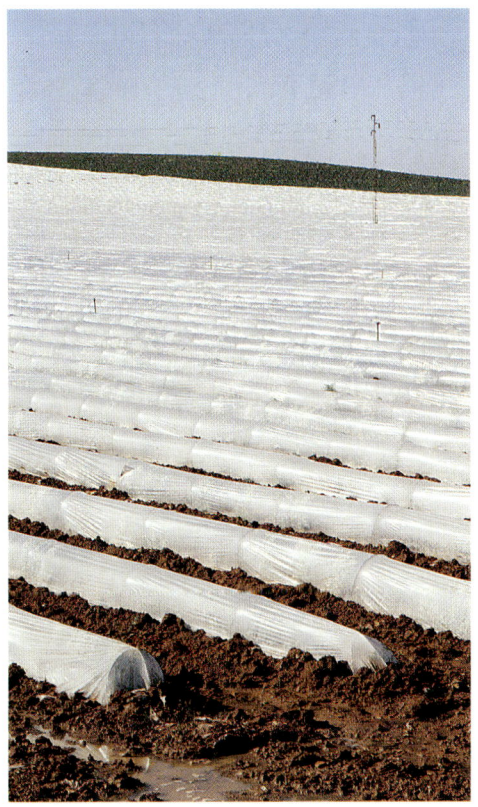

△ **Scientists experiment to produce strains of plants which can resist disease or survive in harsh growing conditions. This scientist is experimenting to find out if mushrooms will grow in wood shavings.**

as if they were factories themselves. Instead of hens pecking around in the farmyard, the birds, known as battery hens, are often kept in crowded sheds with controlled lighting and feeding. The world of the factory has also moved out to sea. Large factory ships now sail with the trawler fleets, processing the huge catches.

Not all these changes have been for the best. On battery farms, animals have often been treated cruelly. Chemicals intended to kill pests on farm crops have actually poisoned wildlife and even people. Factory ships have over-fished important breeding areas often killing other sea creatures, like seals, needlessly.

Nevertheless, scientists today are tackling the same kind of problems as the first farmers did thousands of years ago, but they are now able to produce dramatic results. They design huge irrigation schemes which can make it possible to grow crops in the desert. They breed new strains of plants by treating the seeds with X-rays and chemicals. They protect animals from disease with new medicines.

△ **These plastic covers protect plants from the wind. They also trap precious moisture and maximise the effect of the sun.**

15

Processing food

Some crops are ready to be eaten as soon as they are picked. Apples or tomatoes may need ripening or washing, but they do not need to be processed. Other crops however may need to be treated, cooked or mixed with other foods. For example, wheat must be milled to make flour. This must be mixed with water, yeast and salt, and then baked, before it can be eaten as a loaf of bread.

Much of the food we eat is prepared before we buy it. It may look very different by the time it is sold. When margarine was invented, in 1889, it was made to look like butter. It is really made from oils which have been broken down and mixed with water. The oils may have been taken from food sources as varied as sunflower seeds, soya beans or fish.

Killing off germs

When meat is cooked, it is not just being made to taste better, it is being made safer to eat. Foods contain small living organisms called **bacteria.** Some of these do us no harm. The human body contains all kinds of bacteria which help digestion take place. However, some bacteria, such as salmonella, can poison. These germs can be killed

▽ **Milk is pasteurised before it is sold to the public. During the process the milk has to pass through this heat exchanger, where it is exposed to a heat of 71°C for 15 seconds, and then cooled to below 10°C. This kills dangerous germs.**

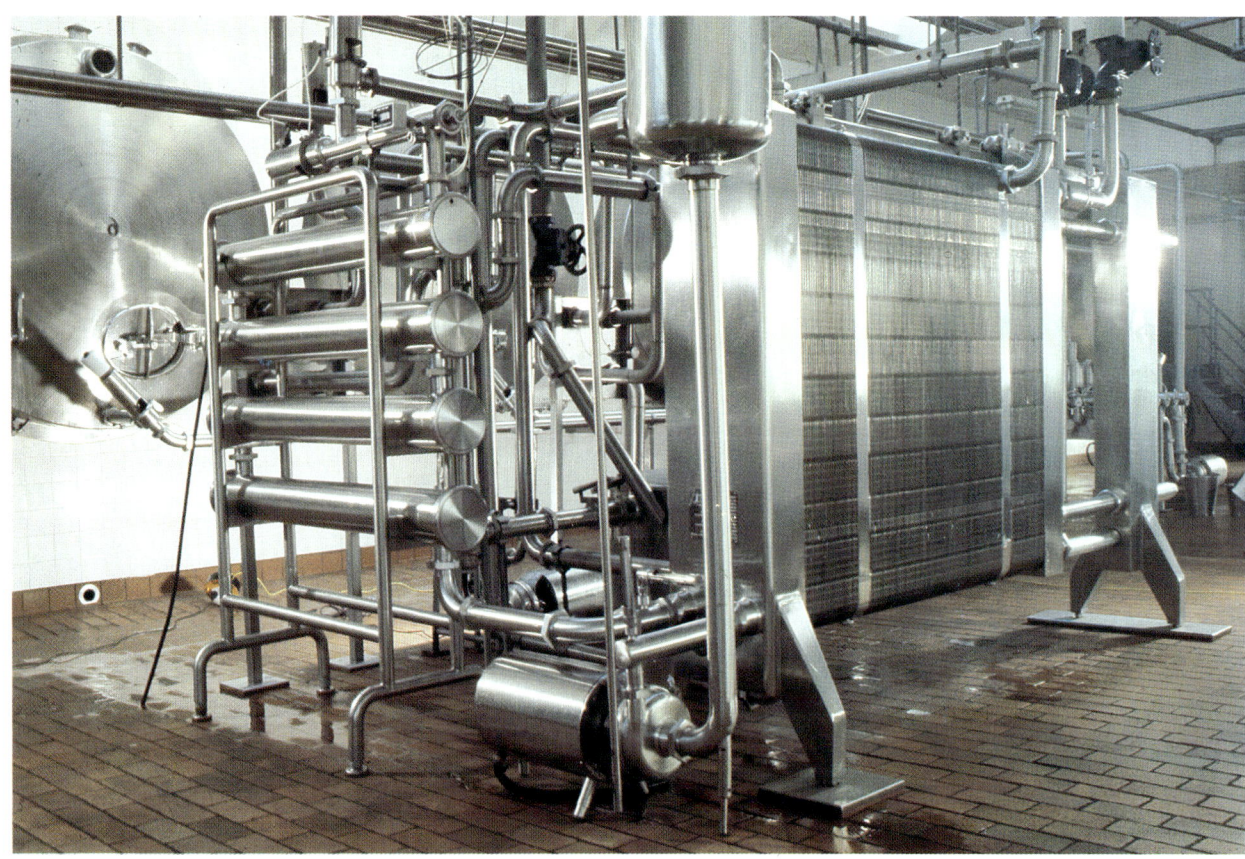

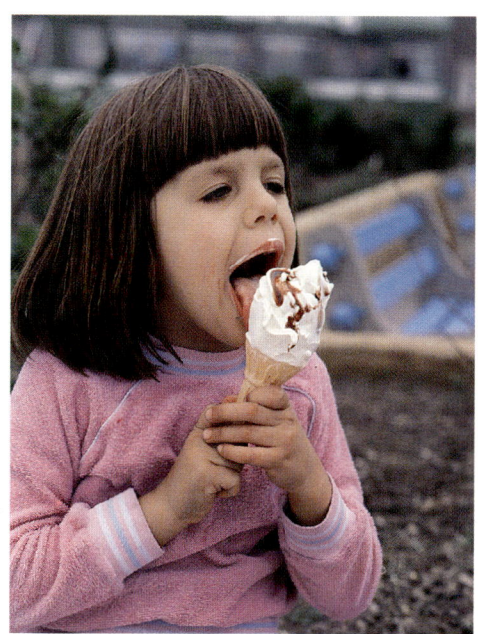

△ **This ice-cream may look delicious and it might even taste good. However, it does not contain any real cream. It is made from vegetable fats, and contains artificial colouring, sweeteners and flavouring.**

by heat, so cooking food thoroughly is important.

Over 100 years ago, a French chemist called Louis Pasteur found that germs in liquids could be killed by high temperatures. Most milk drunk in western countries has been heat treated, or **pasteurised**, first to make sure it is safe.

Adding to food

Today, all kinds of chemicals are added to processed foods. They are called additives. If you look at a packet of food you may see them listed. They include artificial colouring and sweeteners. Flavour enhancers add tastes to the food. Preservatives keep it fresh. Other additives affect the texture of the food, making it stick together or stay firm. Nutrients such as vitimins and minerals may be added to foods such as breakfast cereals, drinks or bread.

The use of additives has meant that packaged food lasts longer, and keeps an attractive colour and taste. However, some additives have been found to be bad for us, and have even been linked to diseases such as cancer. Many people now prefer to buy food which has few or no additives in it. In many countries, manufacturers are now required by law to state on the packet which additives are being used, and whether the flavour is real or fake. Additives have been given standard codes, known as **E numbers**, to help us recognise them.

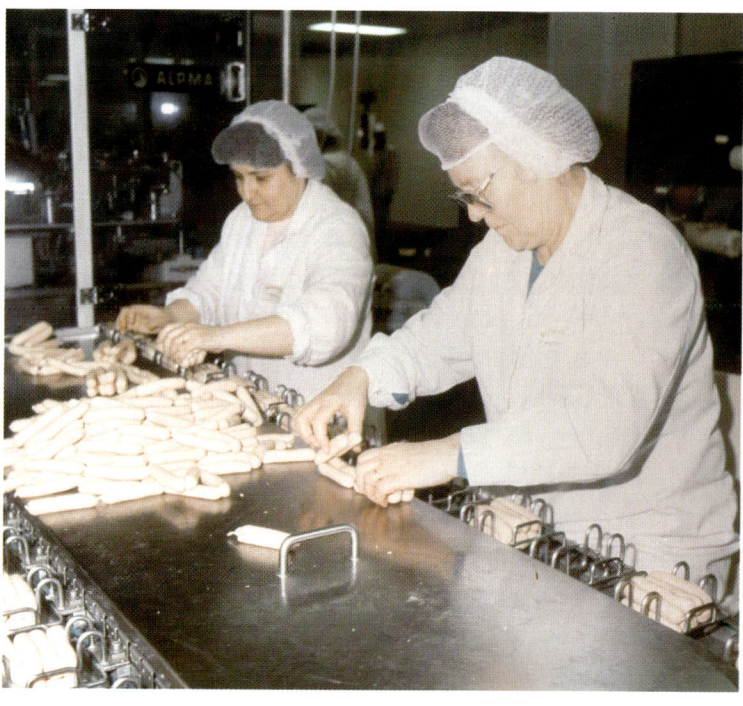

▷ **Many popular meals are made up of processed foods. Sausages are made from minced meat, cereals, salt and other additives. The mixture is forced into an artificial skin, and later cooked.**

Staying fresh

Storing and transporting food has always been a problem. If the store is damp, food will soon go mouldy. Insects may infest flour and other foodstuffs, and rats may steal food and foul supplies. Today, food is stored in sealed containers and kept dry and cool.

The temperature is very important. Many bacteria breed faster when it is warm, and untreated food soon goes bad and decays. Before refrigeration was invented, food could not be kept cold for long periods. Other methods of preserving food were used.

Fresh meat was only eaten in the summer months. In the winter it was heavily salted, or smoked slowly over a fire of wood chips and then stored. Some food was pickled in brine, a mixture of salty water, or in vinegar or alcohol. One of the oldest ways of preserving food was to dry it in the sunshine. All these traditional methods are still used today. We still eat smoked ham and kippers, pickled onions, and raisins, which are sun-dried grapes.

Newer methods

Today, food can be stored in refrigerators. These keep the food cool, and so prevent the growth of bacteria. Many food items, from Brussels sprouts to cream cakes, are deep frozen, so that they can be stored for months. Some people grow and prepare large quantities of fresh food, and store it in their own freezers to eat when the food is out of season.

Bacteria cannot spread if there is no air or water. If food is heated, to kill off the germs, and sealed in an airtight can, it cannot go bad. The metal used in some of the first cans poisoned the food. Today, however, canning is normally safe. The food should remain in good condition and can easily be transported and handled.

Many methods of preserving food are used today. Water can be completely removed from prepared foods such as soups. This drying process is called dehydration. When the food is removed from the packet and mixed with water, it returns to its original state. Other methods include drying by freezing, and cooking and chilling food.

In some countries, food is preserved by irradiation. The bacteria are killed with radio-active rays. This is said to be safe. In other countries, this method is still illegal. There, people fear that this method may cause a loss of nutrients or fail to remove poisons from the food. As yet, there is no

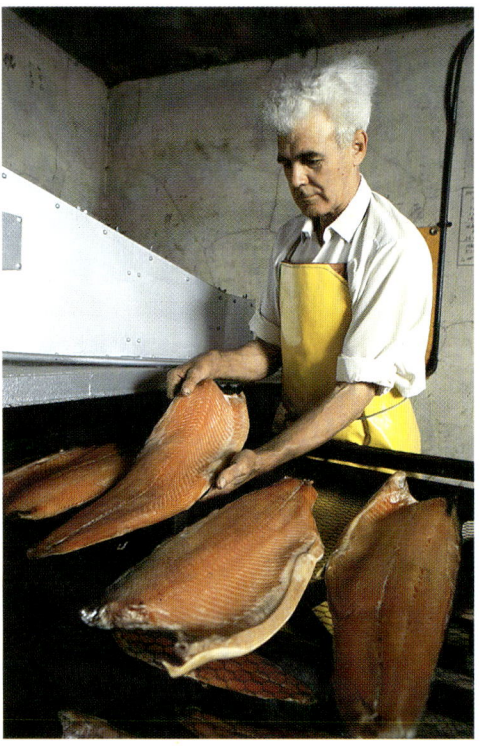

△ Salmon is still preserved by smoking. The fish is salted and then exposed to smoke at temperatures below 19°C. Carbon in the smoke combines with oils in the fish to form a coating which protects it against bacteria. Although we no longer need to preserve salmon in this way, we have come to like the delicious taste of smoked fish.

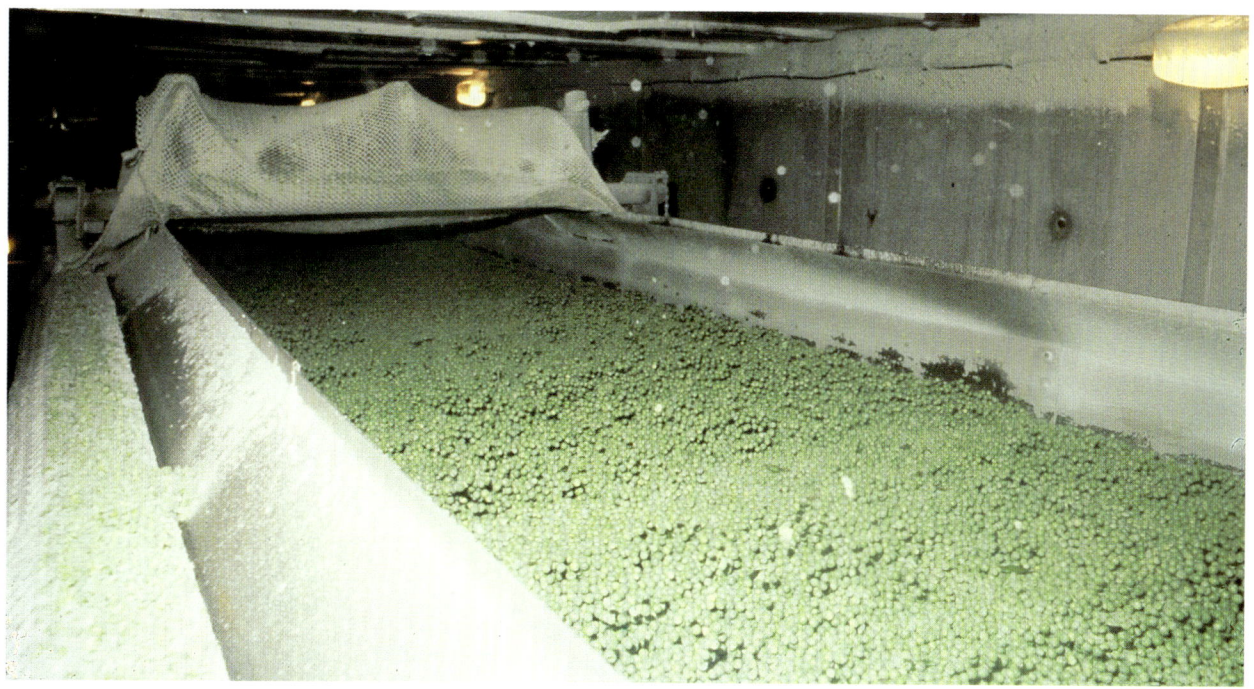

△ Peas must be frozen rapidly, while they are still fresh. As the vegetables pass along a conveyor belt, they enter a wind tunnel. Here, they are blasted with freezing air.

▽ In a canning factory, food is prepared and any sauces or syrups are added. After the food has been put in the tins, air is forced out and then they are sealed. Heat is then used to kill off any bacteria.

reliable way of testing food for irradiation.

Science has not solved all our problems. In recent years, serious cases of food poisoning have been caused by bacteria in eggs, cheese and chilled foods. Farming and processing methods need to be checked very carefully.

Checking on dates

Suppliers of food know just how long it will stay fresh in the shop. This period is called shelf-life. Most food containers are stamped with a date by which the food should be sold. They are also printed with instructions for storing or refrigerating the food once it has been sold.

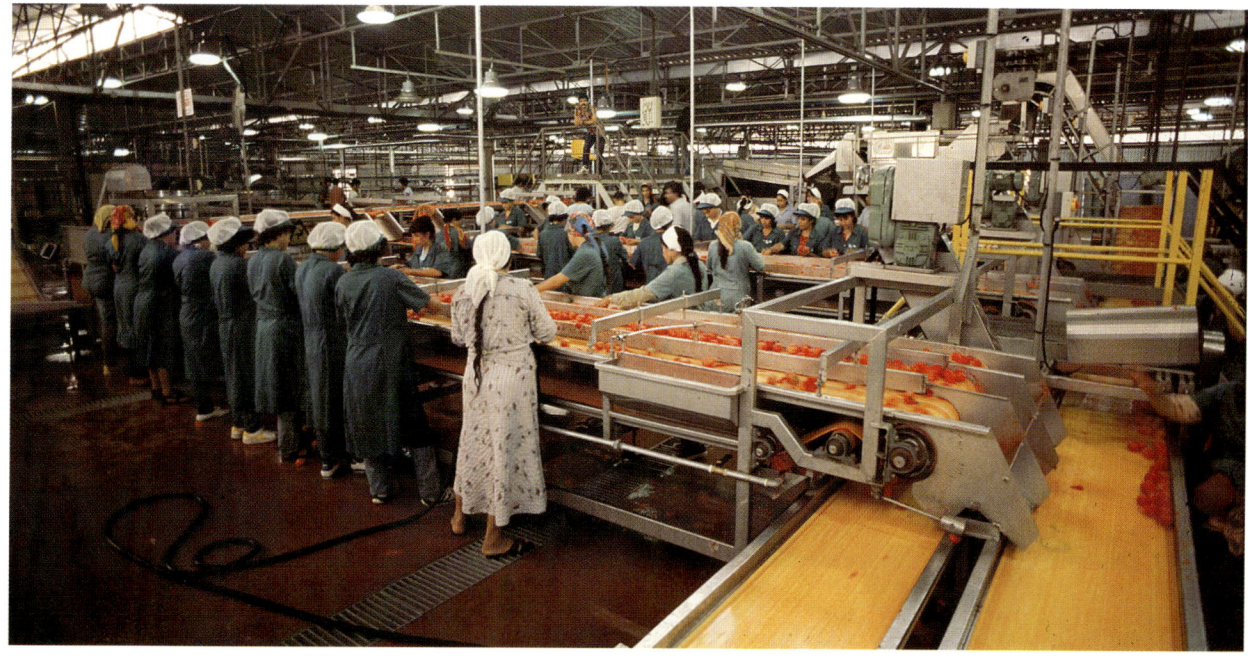

Into the shops

A hundred years ago, most food was sold and eaten in the area where it was grown. Thanks to modern methods of preservation and transport, food can now be exported. Trucks, ships and planes carry canned or refrigerated foods around the world. Europeans can now eat mangoes from Kenya or lamb from New Zealand. Africans can eat canned mackerel from Scandanavia. Some foodstuffs, such as grain, are still transported in bulk. They are poured into the ship's hold and sucked out on arrival. Others are transported in standard-sized containers which can be carried by ship, train or truck.

Buying food

The way in which food reaches the shops varies from one country to another. In some countries, government agencies organize the distribution of food. In others, wholesalers buy food from farmers or importers. They then sell it to the shopkeepers or retailers.

Food is sold or retailed in many ways. There are small shops selling groceries, fruit and vegetables, or the luxury items known as delicatessen. Prices may be higher in such shops, but they can offer a more personal service and more flexible opening hours.

Many towns now have large self-service supermarkets, owned by large companies who can buy food in bulk and use their own storage and transport. This means that they can often sell their goods more cheaply than smaller shops.

▽ **Out-of-town supermarkets allow people to park easily. They can buy a week or more's supply at a single store, and take it home by car.**

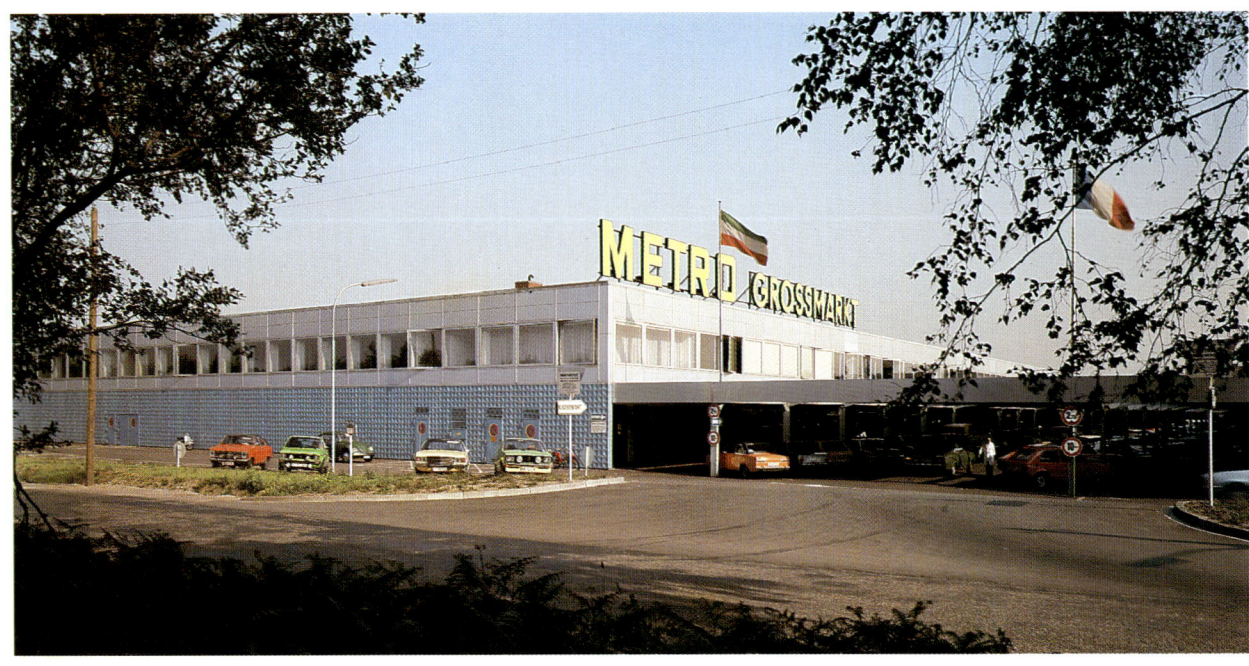

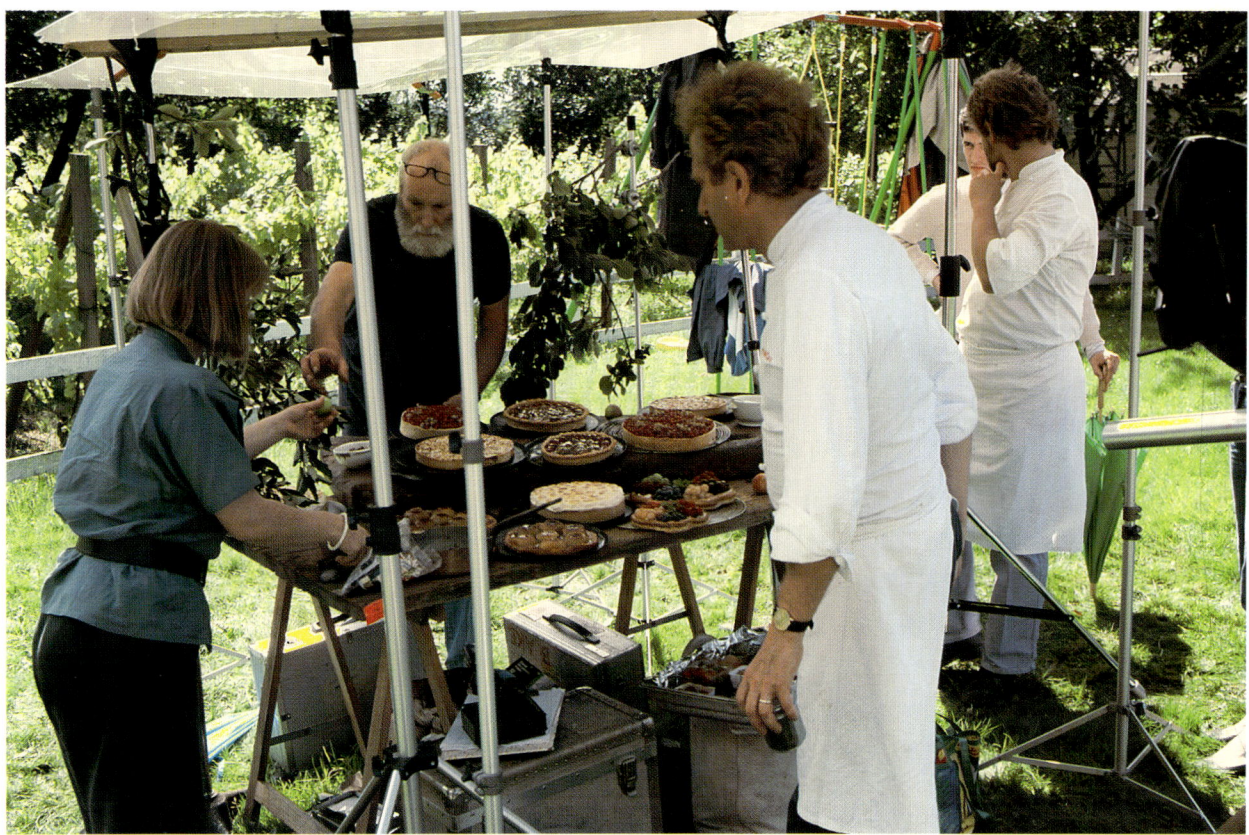

△ **Food advertising is big business. All kinds of tricks are used to make the food look attractive in front of the cameras.**

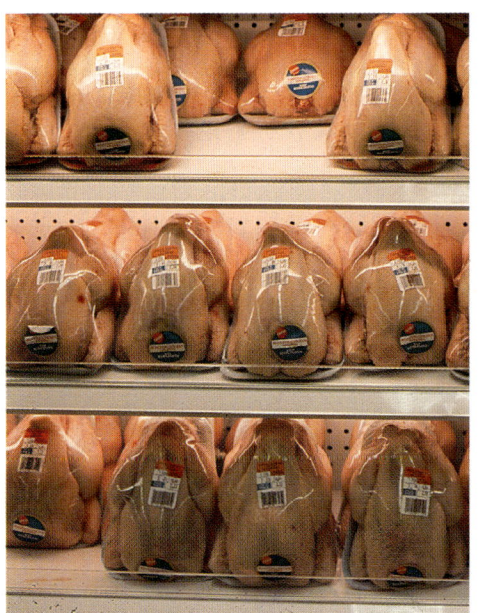

△ **Food must be handled by shop assistants and by customers. Various plastics and foils may be used to protect it from germs. Food must always be stored at the correct temperature and shops should be kept clean.**

Many foods are still sold at open-air markets, especially in countries where farmers still sell their goods locally. Food sold like this can often taste much better because it is very fresh. However, there can be problems because it is difficult to look after food in the open, especially meat.

The food business

Manufacturers and companies spend large sums of money trying to find out why certain foods sell well, and why others do not. They ask people questions, or **market research** a product, to find out about customers' preferences. They advertise their produce on television and in papers and magazines. They make sure that everyone has heard of the **brand,** that is the name of their product. The manufacturers design the packaging of their goods very carefully. Even the colour of a label can affect sales.

We are all influenced by advertising and marketing. We are often persuaded to buy food that we do not really need, such as sweets or crisps. It is important that people remember which foods are healthy. Firms are beginning to take more notice of demands for healthier foods. For example, there are fewer foods on sale now that contain particular kinds of artificial food colouring which are now recognized to be bad for children.

Cooking food

Once the food is bought, it may be cooked in the kitchen of a home, a restaurant or a hotel. It may be turned into a snack or into a magnificent meal. It may be baked, fried, boiled, roasted or eaten raw.

Around the world

Cooking has become far more than a means of making food safer or more pleasant to eat. It has become a form of art. The cooking of fine dishes is known as *haute cuisine*. These words are French, and French cooking is recognised as being one of the best in the world. Chinese cooking is considered by many to be its equal.

Each region of the world has its own special dishes. These depend on the food traditionally available in those areas. Indian food is carefully prepared using a variety of spices. Mexican food is served with beans and chillis. The Japanese are famous for their raw fish, and the Italians for their pasta.

Tastes vary around the world. Most Europeans would think twice before eating snake or dog. Many Chinese people would not like the idea of eating cheese, which they would regard as milk that has gone bad and begun to smell!

▽ **These Chinese chefs are preparing jiaozzi, a vegetable filled pastry.**

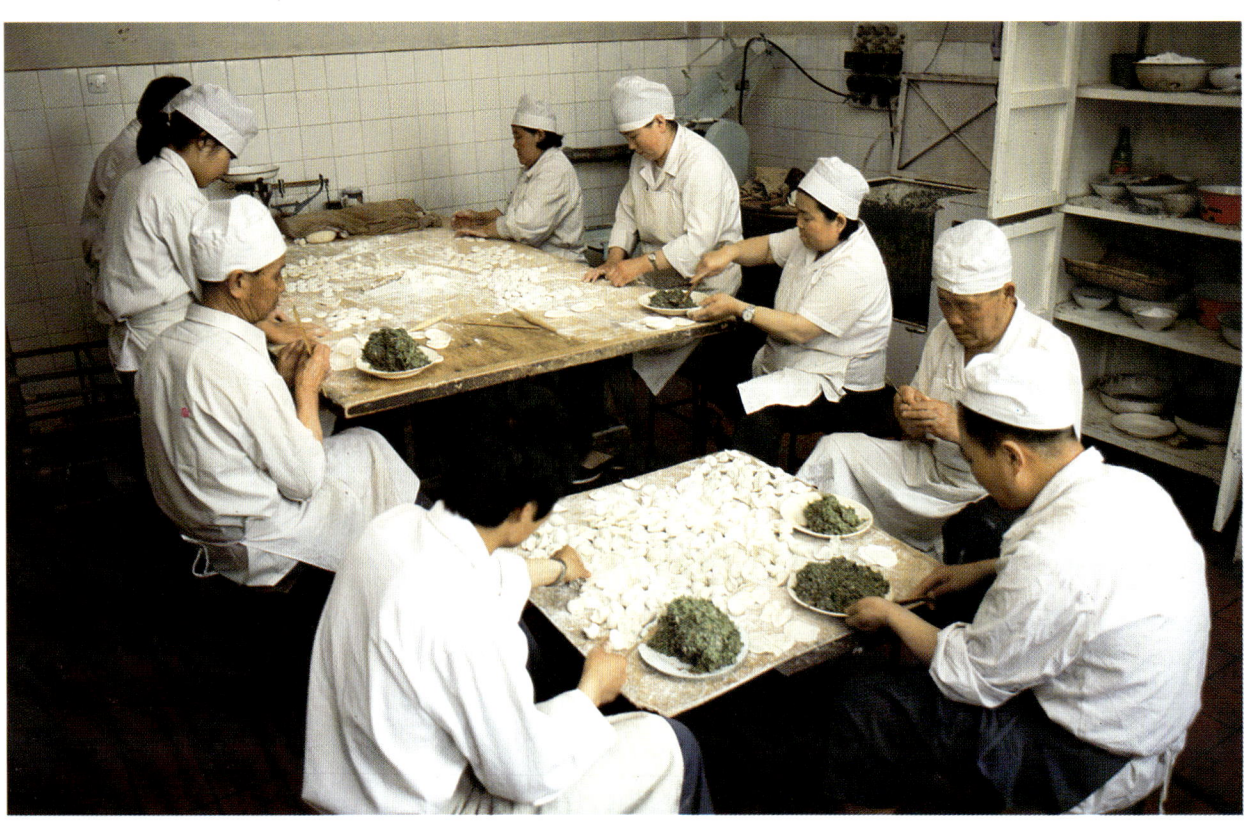

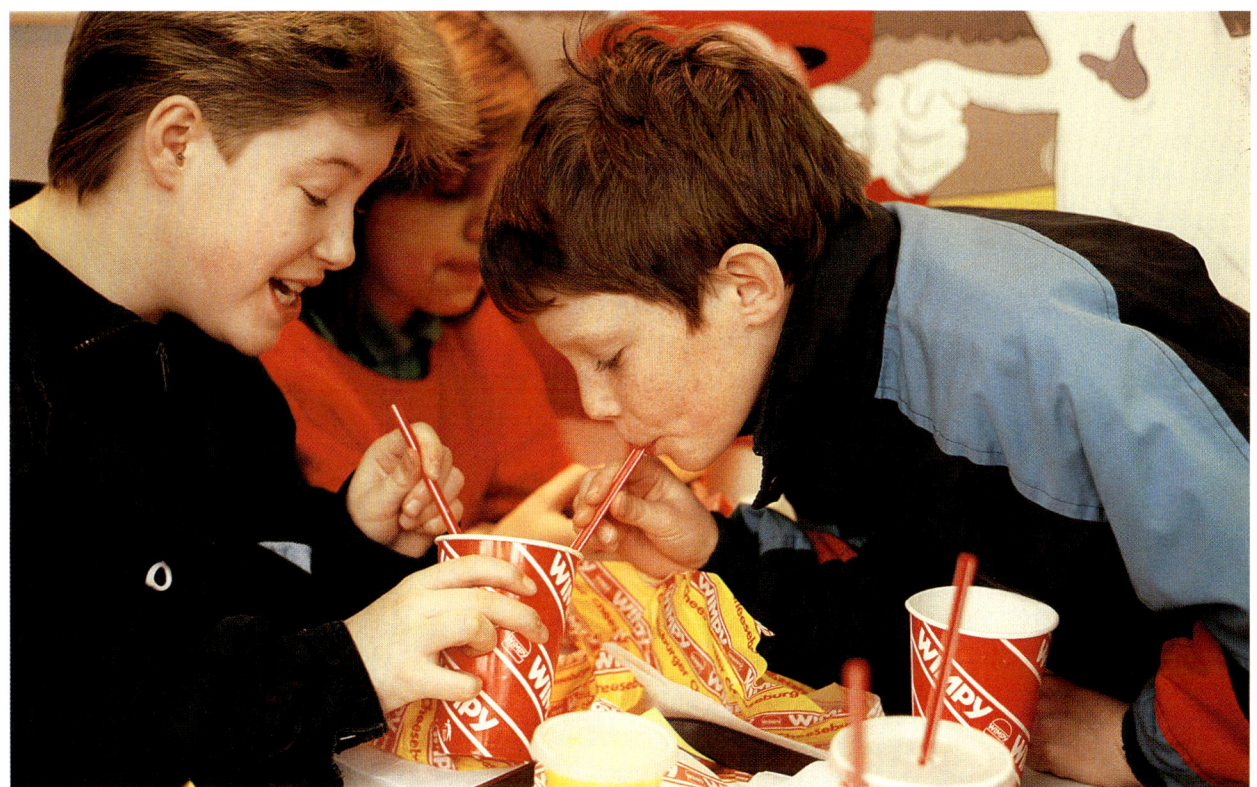

△ Hamburgers provide a quick meal full of protein. However, too much processed and fried food cannot supply all our needs. We need plenty of fresh vegetables and fruit.

△ Gadgets such as food processors make life easier for many cooks today. Work surfaces are easy to clean and keep free of germs. Kitchens must be safe and hygienic.

Instant meals

Modern preservatives, processing methods and packaging have made it possible to provide quick and tasty snacks, such as hamburgers and chips. These are sometimes known as junk foods or fast foods. It is very enjoyable to eat these snacks once in a while, but they do not make up a balanced diet on their own.

Today, whole meals may be bought ready-prepared in a pack. One simply has to boil a plastic bag or heat a foil tray. We all eat such meals sometimes if we are in a hurry. However, there is nothing as good as the flavour of fresh food, which also happens to be much healthier.

Machines and cooking

Technology has changed the kitchen beyond recognition. Food can be cooked under pressure in a tightly sealed pan. Even the toughest meat can be made tender in a pressure cooker, and the goodness of the food is not lost. Gas and electric cookers have made kitchens cleaner. **Microwave** cookers allow meals to be cooked in just a few minutes. They send invisible rays through the food. The rays shoot to and fro at high speed. The tiny parts, or molecules, of water in the food are jostled and heated until the food is cooked. Food processors can slice, grind, blend, mix, and even peel. At the end of all the work, a dish-washer can do the washing up!

To starve or not?

In this book we have looked at the body's need for food, and seen how that food is produced and sold. However, there is a major problem. The system of producing and distributing food does not feed the hungry people of the world. Many farmers cannot grow **cash crops** for sale or export. They can only produce enough food to keep themselves and their families alive. They are called **subsistence farmers.**

Farming and famine

In many parts of the world, subsistence farmers have poor land. They cannot pay for irrigation, fertiliser and drainage. Changes in climate, or over-grazing by cattle or goats can change good soil into desert.

In the Himalayan mountains, forests have been cut down for firewood. This has meant that, as the snow melts and pours into rivers, the water washes away the soil. The result has been serious flooding downstream in Bangladesh. Crops and whole villages have been destroyed.

Trees and hedges also protect farmland from wind and rain. If land is cleared completely so that it can be heavily farmed, the soil can turn into worthless dust. This happened in the United States in the 1930s.

Pests and diseases which affect animals and crops can also cause famine. In tropical areas, swarms of grasshoppers called locusts can strip crops overnight. A swarm can cover thousands of square kilometres and eat hundreds of thousands of tonnes of leaves daily.

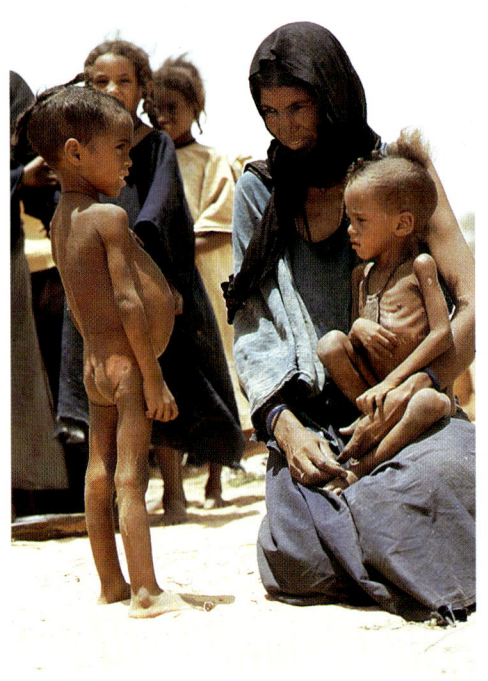

△ **Famine victims often leave their homes in search of food. They need to be provided with clean water, food, shelter, clothing and medicine.**

Rich and poor

In other parts of the world, too much food is produced. Much of it is stored in warehouses and not used. Some may be sold off cheaply. Some is fed to animals or thrown away. Some might be sent to relieve famine, but often there is no point. Butter is of little use if there is no bread.

When famines occur, the richer countries often send food and supplies. The food is usually first transported by plane or ship, and then transferred to trucks which carry it to its destination. It is often very difficult to reach more remote areas. Truck drivers may even find the roads blocked by flooding.

Many people in the richer countries raise money for famine relief. They may organize concerts or hold

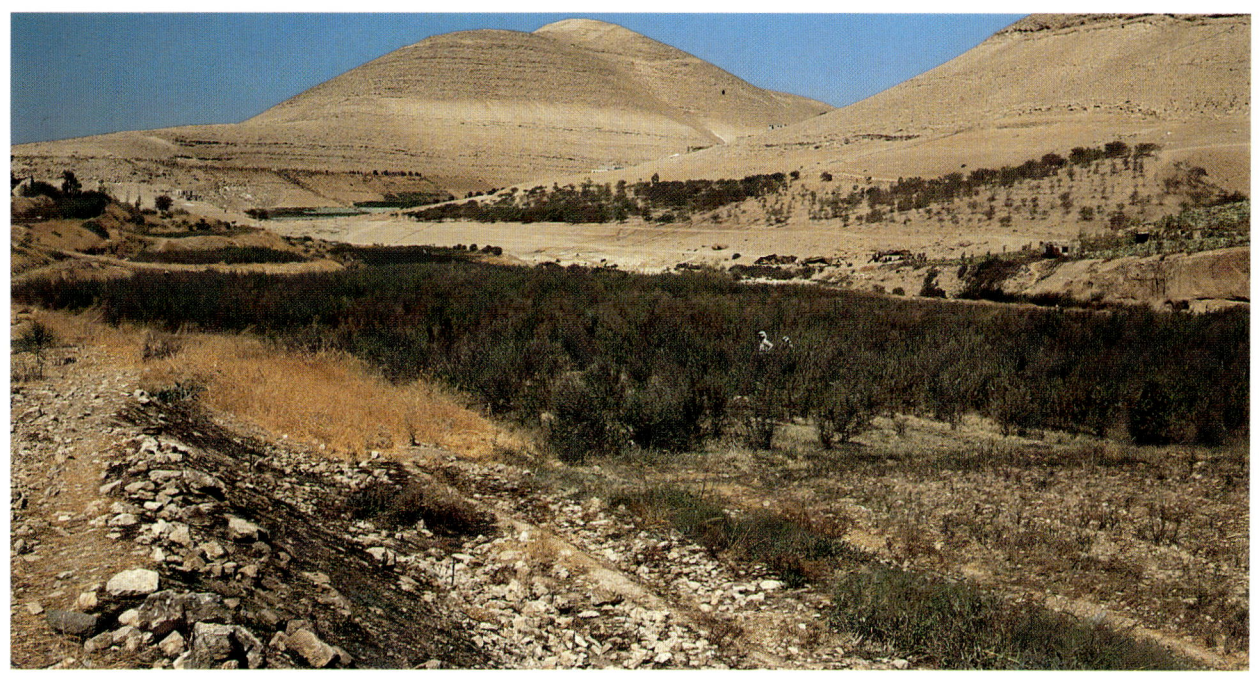

△ **In Jordan trees have been planted to create a barrier against the advancing desert. Trees shelter crops and trap vital moisture.**

▽ **Grain or rice can be shipped into a country, like Ethiopia, suffering from famine. It will provide food for a short time. However, plans must also be made so that there is enough food in the future.**

sponsored events. In an emergency, charity can save lives. However, the money is best used on long-term projects which will prevent famine from happening. For example, trees can be planted so that soil does not blow away. Crops suited to special conditions can be developed. Projects must always be realistic. There is no point in sending out new tractors if spare parts cannot be supplied. Local farming skills and traditions must be developed and not destroyed.

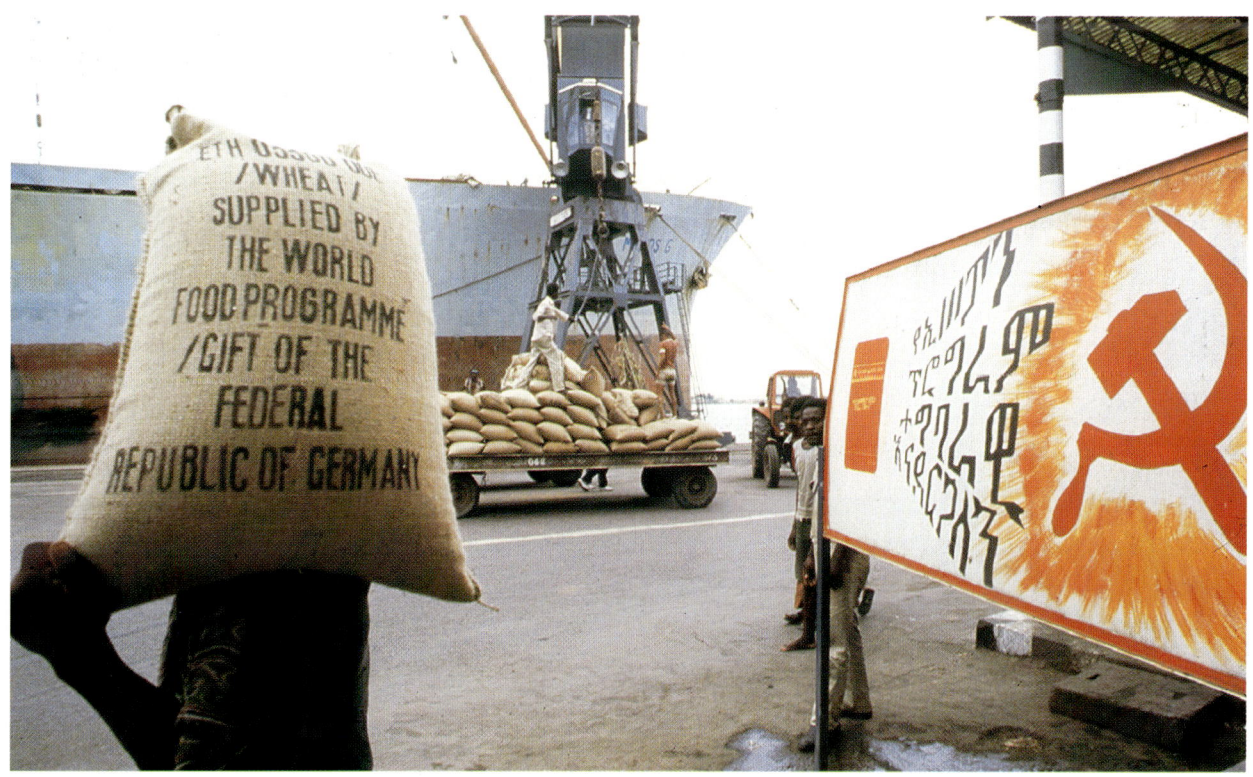

Making sense of farming

The problem of feeding the world's growing population is so important that it is necessary to try to change the way land is farmed. It may be essential to change the whole way in which society is organized and the planet is used.

A small world

The world is becoming crowded, so the best possible use of the land that is available for farming must be made. Raising cattle is a wasteful way of providing food. Crops are grown and harvested, and made into cattle fodder. The fodder is fed to cattle, which continue to graze large areas of land that could be used for crops. The cattle are then killed and prepared for eating. A crop such as soya, on the other hand, only needs to be harvested and processed. A hectare of soya can provide 22 times as much protein as a hectare of land used for raising beef cattle.

The prairies of North America are some of the most productive wheat-growing areas in the world. Much of the world depends on grain from there. However, there are crops easily grown in the tropics, such as cassava, sorghum and millet. These are the crops that can be grown where the world's hot deserts are swallowing up good farmland. Famine must be fought with locally grown produce, not with imported wheat.

▽ **Protein from vegetables such as soya beans is simpler and cheaper to produce than protein from beef.**

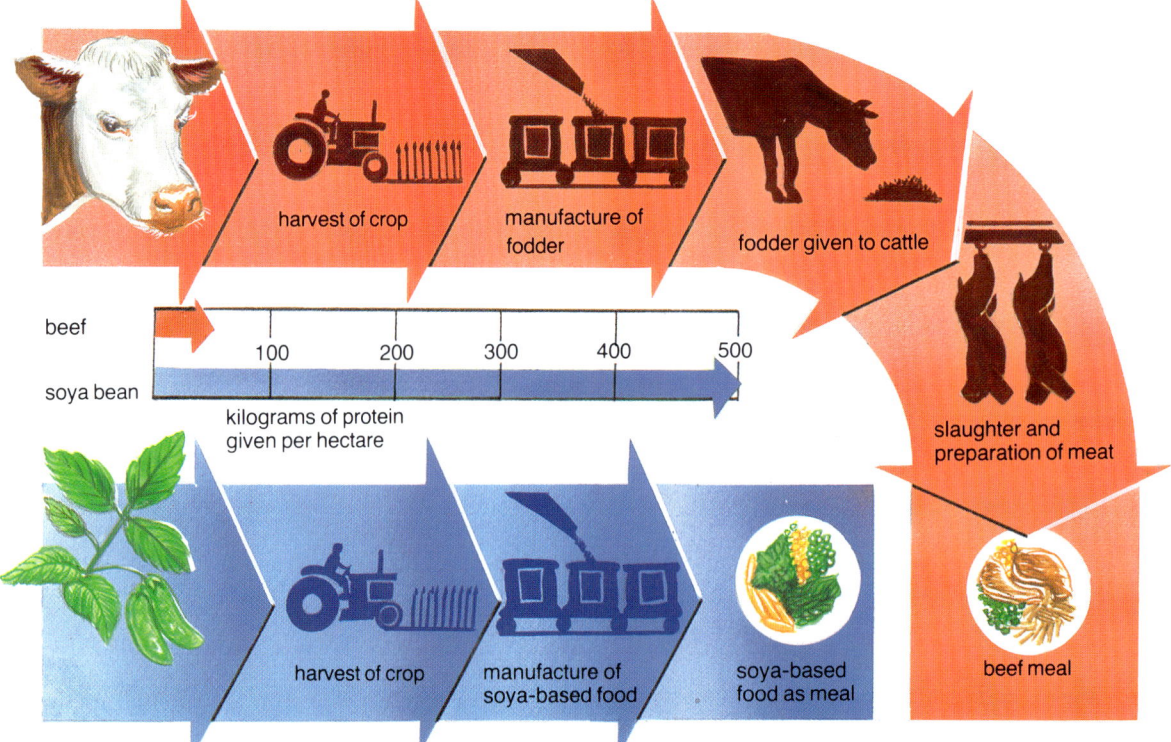

harvest of crop

manufacture of fodder

fodder given to cattle

slaughter and preparation of meat

beef meal

beef

soya bean

100   200   300   400   500

kilograms of protein given per hectare

harvest of crop

manufacture of soya-based food

soya-based food as meal

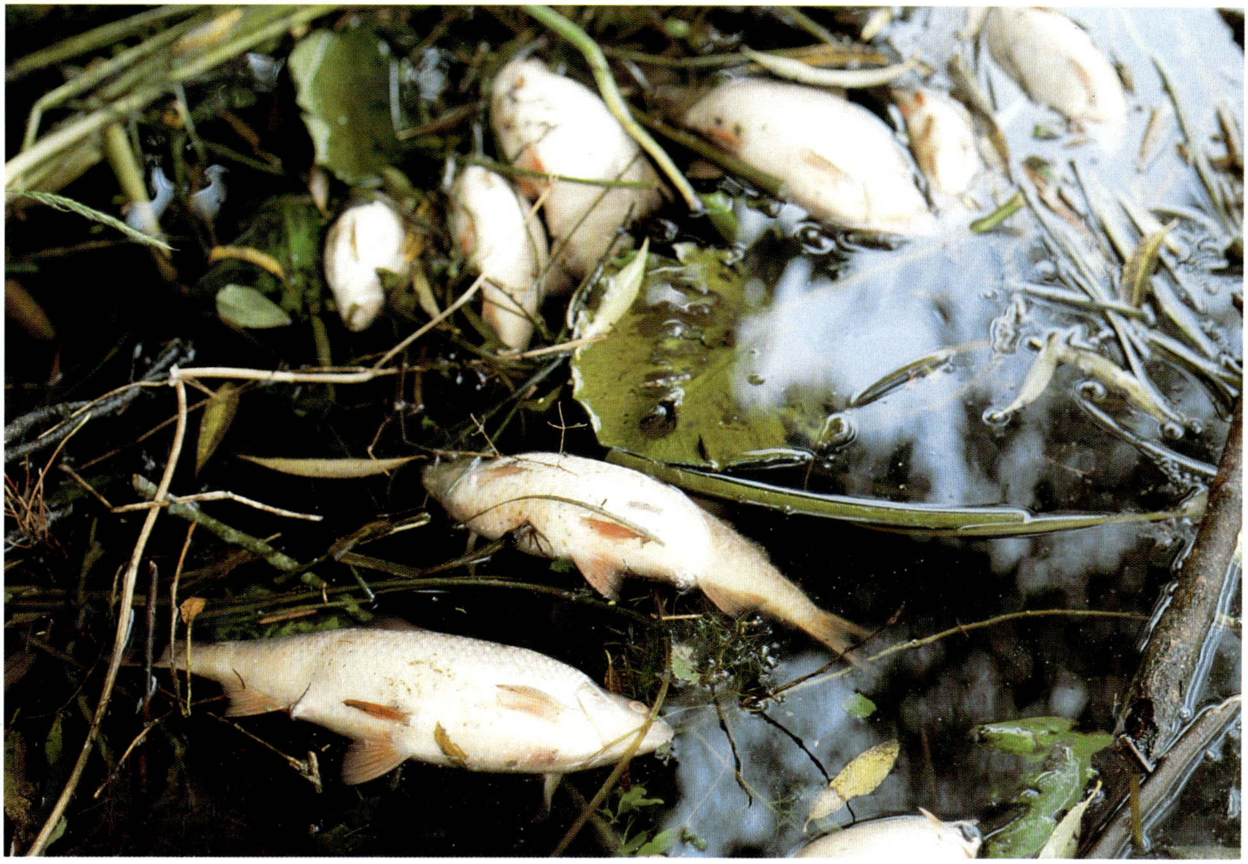

△ **These fish died after polluted farm waste drained into the river.**

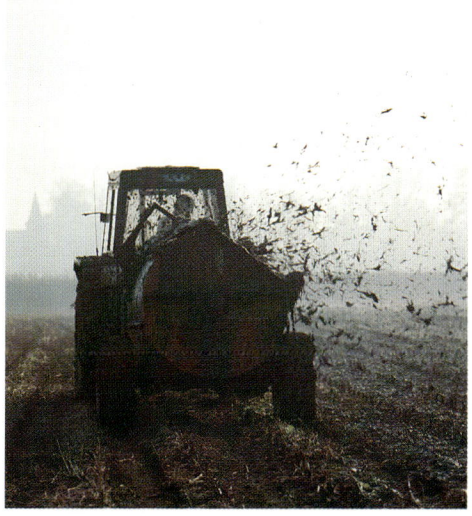

△ **Many farmers do not use chemical fertilizers or pesticides. They use more traditional methods like spreading cattle manure on the fields. The organic foods they produce are more expensive but are preferred by many people.**

Caring for the planet

If enough food is to be produced for everyone, we must look after our planet. Industry has poisoned the rivers and seas. Exhaust fumes from cars have choked the air we breathe. The gases given out by power stations have been carried far and wide by the wind and mixed with the rainfall. This **acid rain** has destroyed whole forests and killed the fish in many lakes.

The pollution of the world may affect the whole pattern of climate. The world may be heating up to the point where the ice caps around the Poles will melt. Scientists have discovered that ozone, one of the gases that form a protective layer around the planet, has been destroyed by chemicals such as those used in aerosol sprays. Scientific farming methods have themselves helped to pollute the planet. Chemicals such as DDT, intended to kill only pests, have poisoned many other creatures, including humans. The clearing of forests for farmland has also created problems. The world's great rain forests, such as those around the Amazon River in South America, provide life-giving oxygen. However, they are being destroyed at the rate of 40 hectares a minute. It is not possible to farm a world that has been turned into a lifeless desert.

One hundred years from now

The search for new sources of food is as important to us today as it was to the first hunters and gatherers of food. Today, however, it is not just one group of people whose survival is at risk, but the whole human race. Now it is the scientists who lead the search for food. They may look at kinds of food that have not yet been used. Twenty-first century fast-food restaurants may well serve worm burgers, with relish made from mould or seaweed! Artificial or **synthetic foods** may be made from petroleum or from recycled food waste.

Scientists are already learning more and more about the way in which animals' bodies work. It is possible to make laboratory copies or clones of animals from a single cell. It is also possible to control the way in which an animal's body grows or how great its yield of milk is. The coming century will see a bitter argument about the rights and wrongs of **genetics**, the science of breeding.

New farmlands

Scientists are already looking for new places to farm. Over two-thirds of our planet is covered by ocean. At a seabed base 100 years from now, visitors might see fish farms,

▽ **This scientist is cloning a plant by cutting up a healthy branch into very small sections. All the sections will eventually grow into a plant exactly like their parent.**

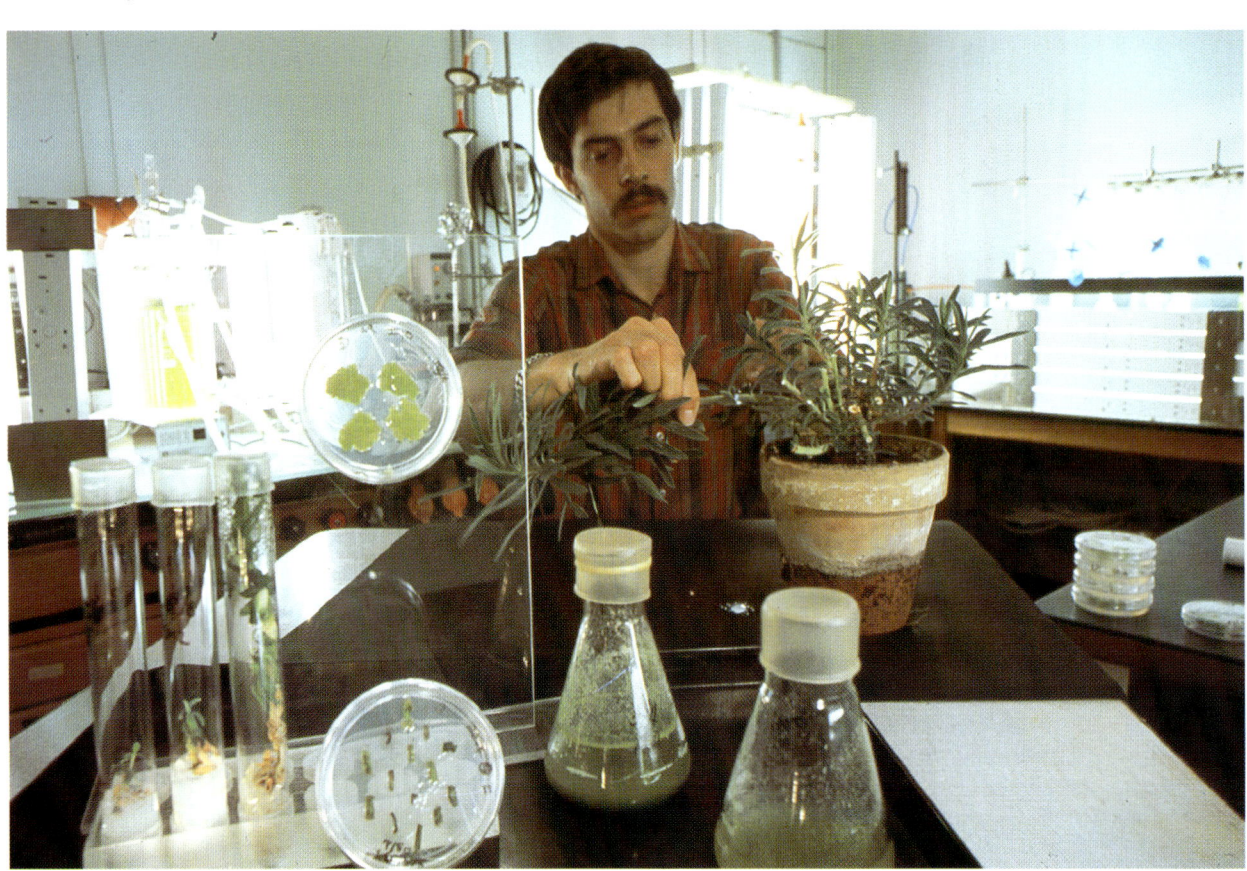

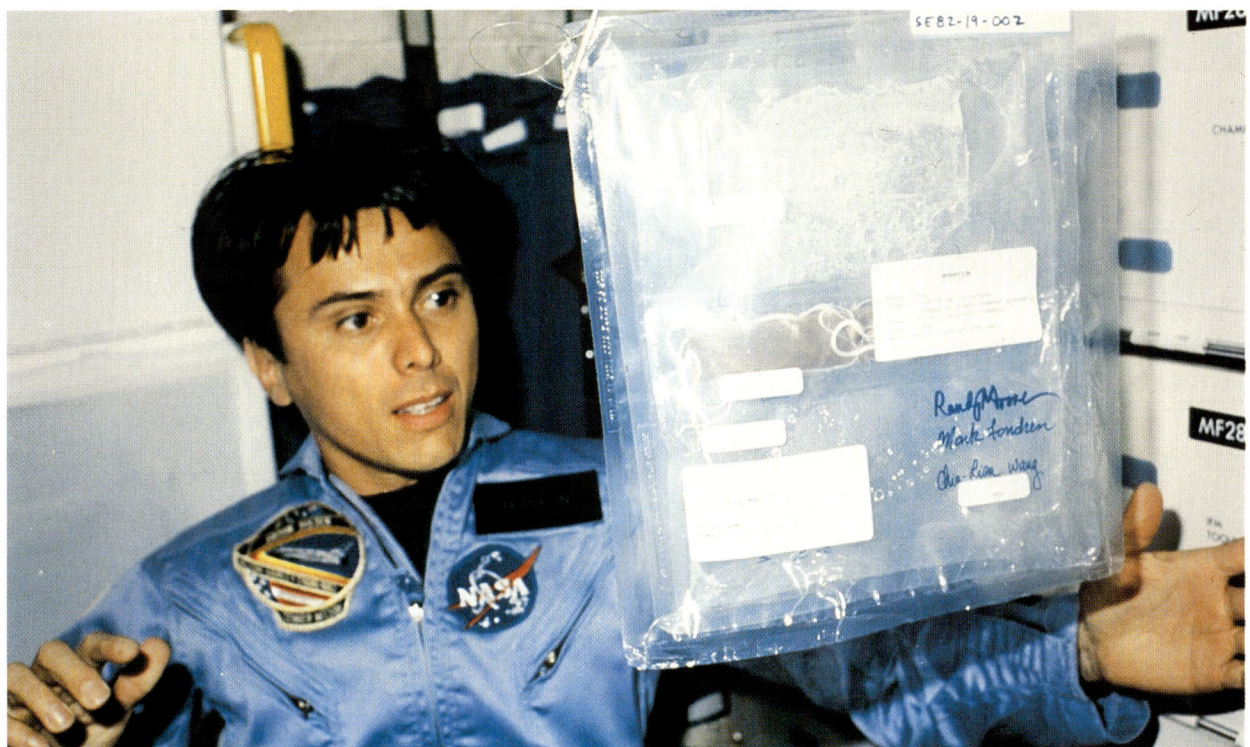

shellfish breeding cages, and fields of seaweed being harvested by submarine tractors.

Seeds have already been grown on board spacecraft, and it is quite possible that in the future large space farms may feed colonies of people. There is sunlight in space, but there is not water or air. These will have to be supplied artificially if crops are to be grown. Farm modules could form parts of a spacecraft or part of a land base built on another planet or moon.

Climate control
It is already possible to make it rain by using aircraft to drop various chemicals into clouds. This is known as **cloud-seeding**.

Other methods of controlling climate may be used in the future. Rivers, lakes and even seas may be diverted to make barren lands warmer or wetter. The icy climate of Siberia could be altered in this way. Scientists however have warned that interfering with nature on such a vast scale could be dangerous.

Health and the future
Medical science will continue to find out about the way that nutrients fuel our bodies and keep them healthy. Food related illnesses such as heart disease should be much less common in the 21st century. New diets will be worked out that really do keep us healthy.

△ **Seeds sprout in space. This experiment was carried out in Skylab in 1986. Scientists wanted to know how plants grew when they were not affected by Earth's gravity.**

The way of the future

Today, there is the microwave oven, the process of irradiation and there is the technology to grow plants in space. However, there is little point in making science fiction come true if scientists cannot come up with inventions to help the subsistence farmers of Asia and Africa in their struggle against starvation. Some engineers are concentrating upon **intermediate technology.** This uses simple materials to make machines which are cheap and easy to run.

Simple inventions

There are many examples of ways in which problems can be solved. One is that African cooking stoves could be examined to find out how they are traditionally built. If they can be made more efficient, they will use less fuel. If less firewood is needed, fewer trees will be chopped down. This will save farmland from the desert.

Improving the design of village waste and compost tanks will help to fertilize the fields. As well as giant combine harvesters, the world is in desperate need of mini-tractors and threshers which are reliable and cheap to run. The key to success is to think of inventions which save energy and which can be successfully worked by the villagers themselves.

Food processing too is often best organized on a local scale. Why build a huge central factory to process sugar cane when a smaller local mill can be built for less money? It is possible that the inventions of the past will help us to use the advanced technology of the space age in a more productive way in the future.

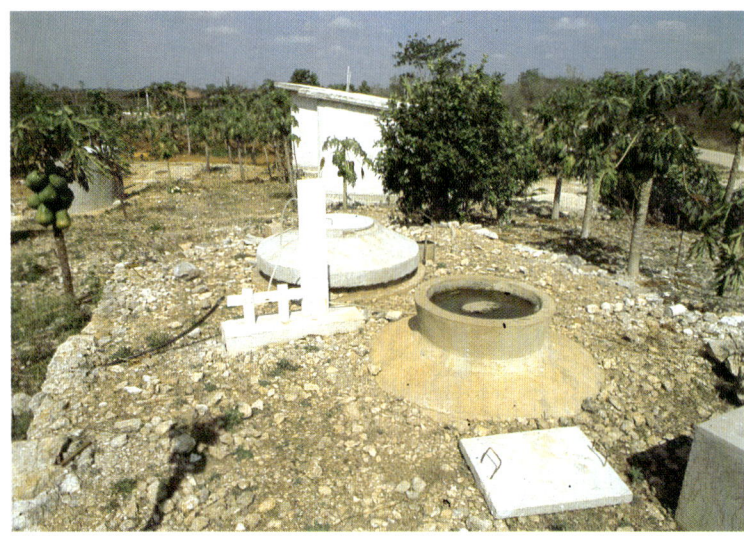

◁ **Human, animal and plant waste are put into this waste tank. Bacteria break down the waste into liquid manure which can be used as fertilizer on the fields. A by-product of this process is methane gas which can be used to generate electricity.**

Glossary

acid rain Rainfall that is mixed with chemicals, particularly sulphates, and pollutes the air. It destroys plants and fish, and can even cause stone buildings to crumble.

amino acids Chemicals found in proteins which are broken down and rearranged in the human body. The acids give us energy and repair our cells.

bacteria The simplest living organisms. Bacteria which spread disease and make food rot are known as germs. Other bacteria help the digestion of food.

brand The name under which a product is sold.

carbohydrates A group of chemicals found in plants, which provide humans with food. They include sugars, such as those found in sugar cane and beet and in milk and fruit. They also include starches, found in potatoes and cereals.

cash crop A crop grown for selling. The farmer lives on the money he makes from the sale.

cell Cells are the building blocks of all living things. The human body is made up of about 50 billion of these tiny units. Each one processes the goodness it receives from the food we eat and carries out its work of keeping us alive.

cereal Any grass-like plant producing grain, such as wheat, barley, oats, rye, sorghum, millet, rice or maize. The term is also used to describe prepared breakfast foods.

cloud-seeding Making rain during a drought by dropping chemicals, such as carbon dioxide and silver iodide, into the clouds from an aircraft.

digestion The process by which the goodness is taken from the food we eat and passed into the body.

E numbers The numbers given to additives that colour or flavour food.

enzymes Substances produced by living cells which bring about chemical changes. Our bodies produce enzymes such as rennin and pepsin to help us digest the food we eat.

fats Substances found in meat and dairy produce, and in oils made from seeds and nuts. Fats react with vitamins to provide energy and help the body grow.

fatty acids Chemicals released as the enzyme lipase breaks down fats. Fatty acids give us energy.

fertilise To make soil richer by spreading it with manure, compost, or chemicals.

genetics The study of how the characteristics of one generation of plants or animals are passed on to the next generation.

glucose A type of sugar formed by the breakdown of carbohydrates. It is stored in the liver as glycogen and turned back into glucose when needed.

glycerol A substance formed when fats are broken down by an enzyme called lipase. Glycerol is stored in the liver as an energy reserve.

hybrid A cross between two plants or animals of different species.

intermediate technology High technology describes the latest engineering. Low technology is simple manufacture of tools like fish hooks. Intermediate technology lies between the two, using modern theories but only simple and cheap materials.

irrigation Systems of channels or ditches designed to carry water to crops in dry areas.

malnutrition A disease caused by an unbalanced diet, too little food, or digestive problems.

market research The way in which companies find out who buys their products and why.

microwave Describes any ray with a wavelength between 50 cm and 1 mm. Microwaves which travel quickly are said to have a very high frequency. When passed through food they knock against the molecules of water in the food. This makes them hot and cooks the food very quickly.

minerals Substances which the body needs to stay healthy, such as iron, salt, calcium, phosphorus, salt or sodium, and chlorine.

nutrients Substances which nourish living things, repairing their cells and providing them with growth and energy.

pasteurise A system of heating foods such as milk in order to kill bacteria or prevent them spreading.

proteins Chemicals which react with enzymes to produce acids in the human body. We need the protein in the foods we eat in order to stay alive.

pulses Seeds of plants such as peas and beans, which can be cooked and eaten for their high protein content.

subsistence farmer A farmer who grows just sufficient crops to keep his or her family alive.

synthetic food Artificial food made by chemical reactions rather than by natural processes.

vitamins Chemicals which the body needs to function properly. They do not provide energy themselves, but react with other chemicals to fuel the body. Vitamins are not made inside the body. They must be taken in as part of our diet.

Index